Cathy's Weightloss Diary

Volume One
2001 - 2003

Cathy Davies

Cathy's Weightloss Diary Volume One 2001 - 2003

Cathy Davies

Extracted from the popular website
cathysweightlossdiary.co.uk by Neil Davies

C&N Publications 2013

History Of Me

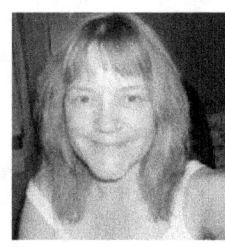 Well... I was born weighing just 2 and a half pounds.

I had asthma until I was 9 years old, quite bad, spent 10 weeks in a 'chest' hospital and had inhalers all over the place (friends, family houses etc)

When I was 10 years old I got IDDM (Insulin dependant diabetes)

I always wanted to be a nurse when I was younger

I have 3 sisters (all younger than me)

Left school at 16 then did a 2 year pre-nursing course at college.

Jobs I have done over the years -

- Summer Playscheme Worker
- Care-Assistant
- Neighbourhood Teamworker
- Chalet Maid
- Shop Assistant
- Clerical Worker
- Opthalmic Technician

Hobbies I had when in my Teens - let me think....I loved reading, I wrote hundreds and hundreds of poems (was very good at rhyming) going to disco's (occasionally), I liked the music but never felt comfy with all the people. I was totally mad on Barry Manilow

When I was in my early 20's I went on holiday to Malta and Portugal, I loved Malta.

In my late 20's I went to college again and did a 2 year Diploma in Psychology and Sociology... I got my Diploma despite a car crash a few weeks before the finals. (I was not the driver and I got compensation).

Late 20's... after college didn't know what to do with myself so to stop mum from nagging I went on a 1 year Office Admin course! Except... I only did 6 months because...

I met my husband (he was the Computer Trainer!!!!!!). He proposed after only 1 week of knowing me! I said YES.

AND THAT'S WHEN MY WEIGHT PROBLEMS BEGAN...

Sorry Neil!

2001

Week 1

Monday 21 May to Thursday 24th May 2001

Went to the gym on Monday! Also went to the gym on Wednesday! Wow aren't I good! Had a takeaway on Thursday night and I ate some ice-cream (silly me!).

Thursday 24 May 2001

11 stone 3 lbs - 157 lbs

Judith came round this morning to get weighed. I had lost 1 lb which I am so pleased about, Judith had gained 1 lb. We have both got to try harder to get rid of this weight. I wore a short pale pink skirt and a lemon top today. I thought they looked ok, thought I looked ok. Went round Tesco in the evening with Neil, we ate there, I had veg lasagne + chips (should have had jacket potato) and on the way home in the car I ate a small bag of malteasers (will I never learn?). We bought a Polaroid film pack and we took each others' photos. I nearly died when I saw mine - I look like a bloody barrel!! I look awful, truly awful. Mind you, Neil looks worse (sorry Neil!). He now weighs around 19 and a half stone (273 lbs), he's about 5 ft 8 inches tall. He won't let me put his pics online. Still, we both did our ab-crunches tonight, Neil does stretches .

NOTES

So this is my first week, I have some way to go. Altogether I want to lose round about 30 lbs. I will have to sort out my eating and do more regular exercise.

Week 2

Monday 28th May 2001

Bank holiday! We went out to a candle workshop. I had ice-cream. Also went out for a meal in the evening (I ate just what I wanted!!!!) We are eating out too much (no wonder we are low in money and not losing)

Thursday 31st May 2001

11 stone 4 lbs (158 lbs)

YEAH. I did so well today. Judith came round and ok so we both put on a pound (what did I expect!), but I made us a great huge salad for lunch and we took the kids out in the afternoon to the park. I ate healthily all day (well... I did have 3 pieces of toast in the evening, but Neil said NO I couldn't have anymore - good job!!)

Friday 1 June 2001

Don't want this site just to be a list of things I have or haven't eaten. Did start dietwatch but got fed up of it cos it was mainly US foods. So if anyone knows of a diet site where I can record my food intake, please email me.

Went to a daytime party today (arggg no food in sight?), had 1 glass of wine, then we went onto a restaurant and I had 2 courses, but J (son) ate most of my 2nd course!

Sunday 3 June 2001

Week 1 11 st 3lbs (157lbs)

Week 2 11 st 4lbs (158lbs)

Well this week I have not lost weight, but then again I haven't tried (at all!)

I wore a new skirt the other day and yes... when I tried to take it off the zip got stuck and I had to pull like mad and broke the zip. The skirt is a size 16 (not sure what this is in US size), I kid myself that this size fits me, but they don't, I fit into them - they are mega stretched. Skirts this size dig into my waist, it hurts. N (hubby) said he calls me his little cannon ball(!!!!), I look at myself in shop windows and see this very round/short/pregnant looking person. YUCK!!!

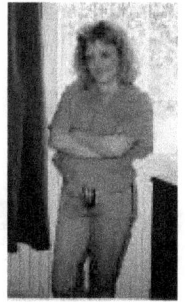

This is me in 1990, I weighed about 8 and a half stone (119lbs).

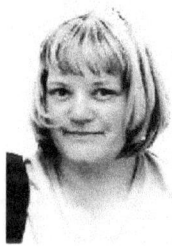

Well, this is me May 2000, I weighed about 10 stone 7 lbs (147lbs), but don't look as fat as now cos of my hair I think?

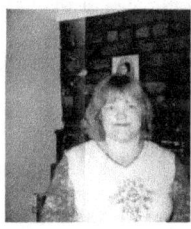

This is me May 29th 2001

Week 3

Monday 4th/Tuesday 5th/Wed 6th

Not too bad, though I did have chips on Tuesday night (something I very rarely have as a rule).

Week 1 11 st 3lbs(157lbs)
Week 2 11 st 4lbs (158lbs)
Week 3 11 st 5lbs (159lbs)

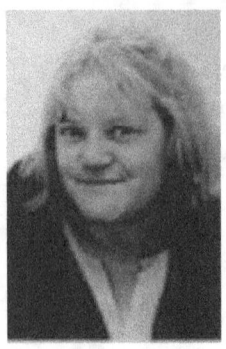

This is me on 6th June 2001 (my body does not go with my head!)I have the wrong body!

Thursday 7th June 2001

11st 5 lbs(159lbs)

Well, I'm just waiting for Judith to come round so we can get weighed. I feel as though I have lost weight (as in, it's not a 'fat day' today). We'll see!!!!!

OK, OK so I put weight on, just 1 lb. Judith came round (she put 2 lb on) and we have both decided that from next week each time we put weight on we will have to put extra money in the tins. NO MORE CRAPPY EATING, NO MORE NIBBLING, NO MORE TAKE-AWAYS.

Week 4

Monday 11th June/Tuesday 12th June/Thur 14th June/Friday 15th June/Sunday 17th June 2001

Went to the gym on Monday. Ate some chocolates (which I didn't mean to do) on Tuesday (and I wonder why I don't lose weight!)

I have decided to write a summary of the week rather than pages and pages of day to day. My weightloss weighing starts NEXT week.

Week 1 11 st 3lbs(157lbs)
Week 2 11 st 4lbs (158lbs)
Week 3 11 st 5lbs (159lbs)

Week 5

Week 1 11 st 3lbs (157lbs)
Week 2 11 st 4lbs (158lbs)
Week 3 11 st 5lbs (159lbs)
Week 4
Week 5 11 st 7 lbs (161lbs)

Monday 18th/Tuesday 19th/Wed 20th June 2001

Went to the gym Monday and did an exercise class (could not do the skipping!). Judith came round on Wednesday and we both got weighed. I am ordering an electronic scales cos it's hard to guess on these.

A NEW BEGINNING

Wednesday 20th June

Today I weighed 11st 7 lbs. Eeeeeekkk!!!!

As you can see I NEED a new beginning cos all my weight has done is go UP. Thursday I did not feel well and slept all day and also I slept all day on Friday (my joints were really hurting and I felt awful, really awful).

Saturday (today) I did some stuff in the house, we all stayed in all day. I did eat some chocolate that N had gone out and bought for the kids. Friday I went to the gym but it was SO hot I only stayed half an hour.

Sunday I went to my mums for the day, did ok eating but when N picked us up later we were hungry on the way home and stopped off at the OK Diner. I had chicken/bacon double-decker sandwich with fries and pancakes.

Week 6

Week 1 11 st 3lbs (157lbs)
Week 2 11 st 4lbs (158lbs)
Week 3 11 st 5lbs (159lbs)
Week 4
Week 5 11 st 7 lbs (161lbs)
Week 6 11 st 4lbs (158lbs)

Monday 25th June to Sat 30th June

Today (Mon) I am going to count points properly and I am going to have JUST 20 points. Nessa (sister) has started Slimming world and lost 3 lbs so far.

I did *not* count points.

Today, Wednesday, I have eaten crappily (as you can see). Once again, I have to keep trying.

Thursday 28th June

Today Judith is coming round and we will get weighed!!

Well Judith came round and we used the new electronic scales (much better). I weighed less, so did Judith. Well done Judith, keep at it!. It makes you feel SO great when you see you've lost weight, even if it might not be quite true cos of new scales!! I had a nice email from Terri in St Mary's Georgia (USA), she (or he not sure) liked my site (thank you Terri). Did some ab crunches (100 in all) and 50 side bends. I keep hearing different things about ab crunches (whether they are any good or not?). My stomach is so yuck, all hanging there and flabby and ripply (courtesy of stretch marks!).

The kids are stressing me out (they are both fighting) and I am just in the mood to raid the kitchen (stuffing myself would make me feel better, ease the stress - for a short time anyway).

Can someone tell me why we, 'I', pig out? I went to Tesco and bought loads of fruit (good, good), I also bought 3 low fat chocolate trifles (162 cals each). I ate 2 donuts (mini that I'd bought for the kids - well we all had 2 each!). I nibbled on the grapes (that's okay). But I mindlessly ate the 3 trifles one after the other. WHY? WHY? WHY? Tomorrow will be better. Better had be anyway!!!!

Friday 29th June

I have eaten better today though it's only 4pm and I am fed up of fruit!! Spoke to Judith on the phone - try and have less wine Judith!. On the other hand, you can't give up everything!! I find the evenings hard, I always want to sit down watch telly and eat when the kids have gone to bed. It is so nice to eat something you really want when you are watching telly. It's no good having veg or fruit then, that's just so yuck at night time. I want savoury, sweet, toast (lots), anything yummy!!

Wed 27th June
2 toast/egg mayo sandwich + chips
2 apples
3 bacon + roll
6 jaffa cakes
chocolate nibbles
2 packs crisps
1 bowl cereal
1 bread
42 points
Thur 28th June
Bran flakes+skim milk
pasta + bacon + tomato
1 options drink + nibbles of quavers
(I ate these so quickly!)
few grapes
dry chocolate cereal
2 small donuts
3 low fat choc trifles (bloody bloody hell)
wholemeal roll + meat + 6 pieces toast
45 Points
Friday 29th June
Bran flakes+skim milk
veg stir fry + 1 rasher bacon + tomatoes

1 banana + 2 plums + some grapes
1 options drink
1 apple
4 slices small crusty bread + grilled chicken
strawberries 'n' cream (could've done without
the cream)

Week 7

Week 1 11 st 3lbs (157lbs)
Week 2 11 st 4lbs (158lbs)
Week 3 11 st 5lbs (159lbs)
Week 4
Week 5 11 st 7 lbs (161lbs)
Week 6 11 st 4lbs (158lbs)
Week 7 11st 3 lbs (157lbs)

SUNDAY 1st July - SUNDAY 8th June 2001

Haven't updated the site this week, I have had mage toothache and J has chickenpox.

WEDNESDAY 4th July

WEIGHED MYSELF today and I have lost a pound!!!!!! So now I am back to what I was in week 1 (I try not to think about it too much!!). How in 7 weeks I have gone from 11st 3 to 11st 3?

Thursday 5th July

I went to friends little girl's party and had a few small nibbles, nothing too bad.

Friday 6th July

I had a root canal filling. But later on in the night I still managed to have almost 3 magnums (ice-creams)!!

Saturday 7th July

My blood sugars are high cos of what I ate last night, I must try and eat better today. It is only 3 weeks till we go on holiday. I bought myself a nice dress from Asda.

SUNDAY 8th July

Felt ill today, have toothache (had root canal!). Have started putting my food into a points calculator/food diary in Excel (sounds good!). I have been slobbing around all day in my pyjamas and have not eaten too much.

```
                Breakfast
        wheat cereal + skim milk
                1 banana
                  Lunch
2 wholemeal bread + tuna + light mayo
                   Tea
        Cornflakes + skim milk
   Extras-1 options drink, 5 rollos
```

Week 8

Week 1 11 st 3lbs (157lbs)
Week 2 11 st 4lbs (158lbs)
Week 3 11 st 5lbs (159lbs)
Week 4
Week 5 11 st 7 lbs (161lbs)
Week 6 11 st 4lbs (158lbs)
Week 7 11st 3 lbs (157lbs)
Week 8 11st 3 lbs (157lbs)

Judith has not been round cos of J's chickenpox - come back soon JUDITH!

Tuesday 10th July 2001

Last night I was so fed up just before N came home, I rang Pizza Magic for a takeaway and we (I) ate a burger + fries and a small garlic bread (ok, ok, silly of me) but to make it worse I took some cream donuts out of the freezer that N had bought (not me!) and defrosted them then ate 3 of them one after the other. Pig or what!

Today I am going to REALLY try harder to eat better. I am aiming to go to the gym this afternoon for an hour

Wednesday 11th July 2001

Well I STAYED THE SAME weight today, which I am pleased about. I mean, I wish I'd lost weight but staying the same is so better than putting it on!

I bought some tablets to help you slim (herbal) off the internet sometime ago, they came the other day. They are called ZOTRIM and you take 2 before you eat (with lots of water). I took some before brekky this morning. I AM GOING TO EAT A HEALTHY DIET TODAY.

MESSAGE FOR N!!!!!!!!!!!!! PLEASE DO NOT BUY ME ANY MORE SWEETS TO EAT AT NIGHT (I HAVE NO WILLPOWER!). STOP BUYING THEM FOR US. STOP.

Thursday 12th July 2001

YES! YES! YES! YES! YES! YES! YES! YES! YES!

I did it, I managed to get through a day without crappy eating, aren't I good! Sad, yes I know, but getting gooder!! (ha ha)! Have I nothing better to do?? Doing this website helps me not eat so much (ermmm...well is beginning to), it's my hobby and I enjoy it (gotta get a life!!?).

I have eaten well today (i.e. healthily!) Dunno if it's all in the mind but since taking the Zotrim, well, I haven't wanted to eat as much??????? We'll see!!! ERrrmmmm... So OK I spoilt it in the evening. I think really it's best to go to bed at 9pm (sorry N!) to avoid night time snacking.

FRIDAY 13th July

Arrgggg! No I am not superstitious!! I am going to do some exercises later. Gave N a huge bunch a grapes to take to work (he needs to nibble!) I have my plums!!

SATURDAY 14th July 2001

Well, it was well and truly Friday the 13th yesterday cos I discovered a few blisters on my leg (bites??? NO)

CHICKENPOX - I HAVE CHICKENPOX!

J is just getting over the cpox and here I am worrying that my 3 yr old might get it too, and lo and behold I get it. Went to the docs this morning and he diagnosed cpox. I didn't eat much yesterday, didn't feel too good! GOOD!!

SUNDAY 15th JULY 2001

I have cpox, with 4 cpox spots so far (I think this will be all!), dumb or what! But apparently I am still contagious. Today I have resisted pigging out in sympathy with myself (admittedly it helps when you don't have much food in!), but I could've sent Neil off on an emergency run to the shops, but didn't. I have to admit that yesterday N had bought some cream cakes and I had 3 of them (I hadn't eaten all day - nothing at all!) - so perhaps that's not too bad?

TUE 10th July
Bfast
cornflakes+skim milk+apple
Lunch
ham + 2 slices wmeal bread + shapers bar
Tea
pasta+tomoatoes+pepper+ onion
Eve
malteasers + minstrels + 2 toast
WED 11th July
Bfast
2 shredded wheat + milk
Mid Morn
1 apple
Lunch
Beans on toast
Tea
Mince n gravy + veg + new potatoes
Eve
2 toast
THUR 12th July
Bfast - 2 toast
Lunch - 2 bread + ham + tomato + an apple
Tea - Salad + wafer thin chicken + tbls mayo +
5 rasuemussen crackers + a banana
Extras - pac of candy sticks
Eve snack - (here's where I goofed up!) 4
toast + 2 bowls cereal + 2 packs crisps

I ate this but...

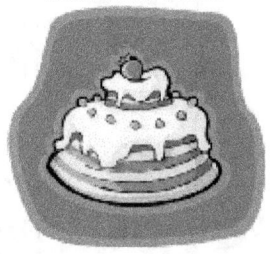

I should've had this!

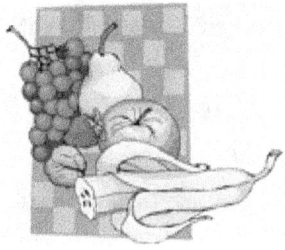

Week 9

Week 1 11 st 3lbs (157lbs)
Week 2 11 st 4lbs (158lbs)
Week 3 11 st 5lbs (159lbs)
Week 4
Week 5 11 st 7 lbs (161lbs)
Week 6 11 st 4lbs (158lbs)
Week 7 11st 3 lbs (157lbs)
Week 8 11st 3 lbs (157lbs)
Week 9 11st 3 lbs (157lbs)

WOW not long for the holiday!

Monday 16th July 2001

Today I have been good (ha ha so far!) sounds silly really... saying oh I've been good... oh I've been SO bad (like, you know, I'm a kid!) I have a blocked nose, it's GREAT, honestly, when you can't smell the food you don't crave it so much! I haven't been to the gym (it's been on my mind though!). When I am not feeling so crappy, being so spotty, feeling so knackeredy... I will pop to the gym when I can (if mother n father-in-law can have the 2 deranged children), since the school breaks up for the summer hols on Friday.

TUESDAY 17th JULY 2001

Had a Chinese this evening (least I've laid off the chocolate!). Now I am so full up I feel sick!!**!! Get weighed tomorrow, can I lose anything between now and then?? Even if I try really hard??!!

WEDNESDAY 18th JULY 2001 GET WEIGHED!

Here I am up at the crack of dawn (well 7.20am), I have already weighed myself (just couldn't wait!).

I have stayed the same, disappointing but I have had a few too many takeaways.

SATURDAY 21st July 2001

Slept almost all of today (my joints are killing me), so NO I am not a lazy so and so!! With the holiday not being far away (and I have not lost the weight I intended) it is a temptation to, well... not bother with trying to diet. BUT, I must keep aiming to eat healthily (less of the diet word)!. Had some shopping delivered from Tesco and yep, most of it was healthy! Have lots of salad and fruit in. WHY do I always EAT when the kids are screaming/fighting and N and I are arguing on and off (all the time!)?? What could I do instead of running to the kitchen????????????????????

SUNDAY 22nd July 2001

Ate brekky at Little Chef (naughty!) and then in the evening N had ordered a Pizza Magic takeaway, we are eating out too often. FAR FAR TOO OFTEN. Here's me saying this and there's a holiday away coming up! BUT I fully intend to do as much exercise as my cronky joints will allow me on holiday, e.g. walking, dancing (?), swimming, swinging on the kids swings in the play area ermm... n stuff like that!

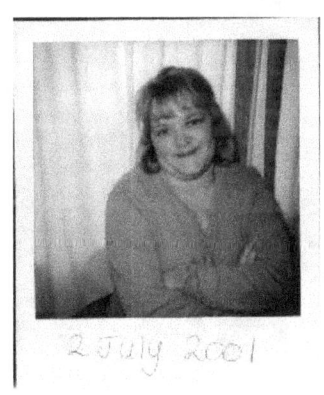

Monday 16th July 2001

```
        Bfast - 2 toast
   Lunch - WW beef sandwich
   Anoon - 1 options drink
```

Tea - Can't remember!

This is no good is it??
MUST GET MOVING ON THIS DIET!

WEDNESDAY 18th JULY

Bfast - 2 toast (3pts)
Mid morn - options drink (1 1/2 pts)
Lunch - 1 wholemeal roll + meat + 1 pack lite
crisps + banana + options drink
(10 pts)
Tea - I roll + meat (3 pts)
I low cake + small buttons (3 1/2 pts)
Snack - snack-a-jacks (2 1/2 pts)
TOTAL = 24 pts

Holiday

Brixham, Devon

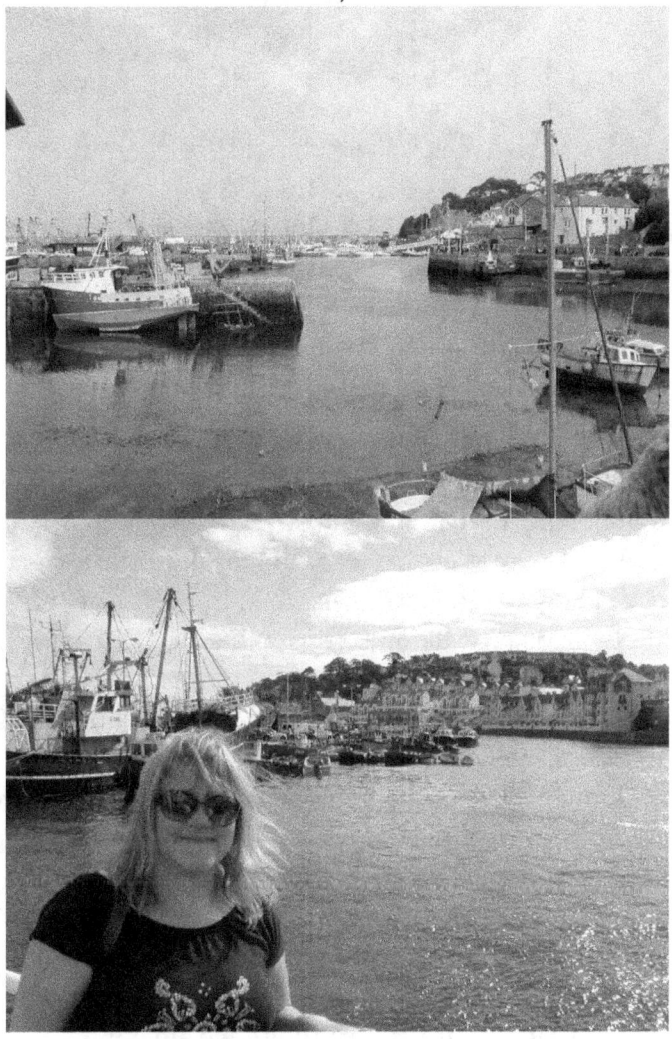

Week 11 - Back From Holiday

Week 1 11 st 3lbs (157lbs)
Week 2 11 st 4lbs (158lbs)
Week 3 11 st 5lbs (159lbs)
Week 4
Week 5 11 st 7 lbs (161lbs)
Week 6 11 st 4lbs (158lbs)
Week 7 11st 3 lbs (157lbs)
Week 8 11st 3 lbs (157lbs)
Week 9 11st 3 lbs (157lbs)
Week 10 11st 2lbs (156lbs)
Week 11 11 st 5 lbs (159lbs

11th August 2001 Saturday

I have just got back from holiday today. I have had 2 weeks of having a great time (mostly!). We went to Brixham in Devon. I had lots of cream teas, some (ok lots) of ice-creams and we ate out almost every meal. BUT, we also did absolutely loads of walking so this will cancel out some of the cream teas!!!!

I must admit I feel like I have put on weight, but I will wait till Wednesday to weigh myself. On holiday I swam a lot also, and I had a great ride on a speed boat (not me driving!!!). We had a few boat trips. We went to a fairground and I had a go on the Terminator (though when they locked the bar over us my ermmm....stomach was blummin hanging over it (hopefully it just looked like my clothes billowing out!!!!). I went on this ride called the meteor (like a round spindryer, I span around), it was great!!. Although we ate out a lot, I never actually had puddings, or desserts (whatever you want to call them), I saved myself for pink n white cornets as we walked around!!

MONDAY 13th August

Well here I am, now I have to get serious and be more sensible if I want to actually lose this extra weight. It's about time I made a proper effort instead of dilly-dallying around. I looked at myself on some video we took on holiday and I look FAR too big, I really don't like the way I look and I don't feel comfortable at this weight.

I will (I will certainly aim to!)

1 Aim to drink more water

2 Aim to eat more fruit and veggies

3 Aim to move about more and not be so lazy!

TUESDAY 14th August 2001

Can't get settled back into the 'being at home' routine, feel fed up really. Ah well!!

What happened to me counting points???? Well, I keep thinking about going back to it but I don't feel very organised at the moment. I did lose weight when I counted points (a year or so ago), so I will try counting again.

WEDNESDAY 15th August 2001 (Weighing Day)

Oooops! Forgot to weigh myself this morning, so will do it tomorrow. I have decided (last night while I was in bed trying to get to sleep), that I will now count the ww points. I actually have a ww points calculator, so rather than worry about writing food down I will just use the calculator religiously.

I have the photos back from the holiday, there are a few awful ones but on the whole they are good, I am going to scan some and put them on this site. It is my birthday on Saturday!! I will be ermmmmm... a year older!! Last night we had a Chinese takeaway because I could not be bothered cooking. I must try now to avoid takeaways, FAR too fattening.

What was I saying???? Tonight we went down to WK lake and ate Pizza Magic (I had a burger + fries + 2 pieces garlic bread). So....today I was gonna count the points but will NOW do it tomorrow. Things do get in the way and spoil your good intentions. It isn't fair!!!! I will start eating better and TESTING my blood sugars - if I keep telling myself these things often enough, then eventually I will do them?? (I hope).

THURSDAY 16th AUGUST 2001

Weighed myself today.

11st 5lbs(159lbs)

I have put on 3 lbs, not too bad I suppose for a two week holiday?? Just got up (10am) and I am feeling stressed already!

MONDAY 13th August 2001

For brekky I ate a banana and a yoghurt (good!) Mid morn I had a banana, lunch was a pac of micro chips and 3 slices of bread + a diet yoghurt (not so good!) Large glass skimmed milk. 3 small lemon meringue cakes, 3 bread rolls, loads of toast (is there something about me and the no. 3?)

Had some hotdogs on Tue and Wed (ok so they were homemade as in plain bun and frankfurter sausages done in microwave with reduced fat tomato sauce). but I ..well....ate 5 altogether (not in one go!) Have I no control????

Week 12

Week 1 11 st 3lbs (157lbs)
Week 2 11 st 4lbs (158lbs)
Week 3 11 st 5lbs (159lbs)
Week 4
Week 5 11 st 7 lbs (161lbs)
Week 6 11 st 4lbs (158lbs)
Week 7 11st 3 lbs (157lbs)
Week 8 11st 3 lbs (157lbs)
Week 9 11st 3 lbs (157lbs)
Week 10 11st 2lbs (156lbs)
Week 11 11 st 5 lbs (159lb)
Week 12 11 st 7 lbs (Argg!)

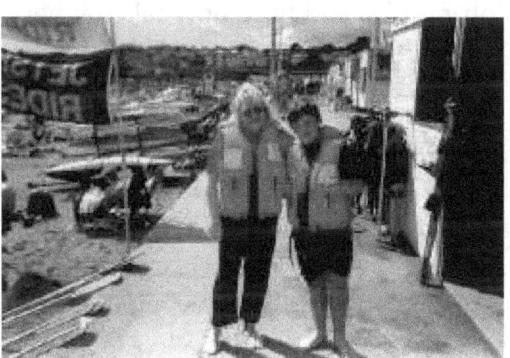

Me and J in Goodrington Sands (Devon) about to go on a
speedboat ride!! Aug 2001

Monday 20th August 2001

I have done a chart to log my water (as in, I will aim to
have up to 8 glasses of it a day to aid in my weightloss).

My sister had a baby girl, they have called her Amie, she
was born yesterday weighing 6 lbs and 2 oz, we will go and
see her next weekend at home. I am really going to start to
make an effort to lose this weight, to eat better. I'm jealous of
my sister (!) cos she has lost 13 lbs with Slimmers World (not

the sister who just had the baby). Judith has said she will 'start' again when the children go back to school on Sept 4th. It is difficult to think about yourself (what you're eating etc) when the kids are off school - you are more tempted to eat 'on the move', pick more and head for the kitchen when they stress you out!!

THURSDAY 23rd August 2001

OK, OK, I have one more, just ONE MORE meal to eat out, I am going to the Indian Rest round the corner on Sat night with my friend Nicola. Yes, I went for a meal last night with N, it was my belated b'day meal (just the 2 of us). I know my b'day was on the 18th, so after Sat night, that's the end of celebration type meals (till erm... our anniversary in October). I started taking the Zotrim today (had an email from Aileen in Scotland, she's lost 10 lb so far which is great), so I have paid for this Zotrim (£22) and have only taken it here and there so I should (for it's price!) use if properly in the hope it helps!!! I weighed myself yesterday (very quickly!) and I was 11st 7 lbs, with some clothes on!!! NEXT WEEK I WILL WEIGH LESS!!

SATURDAY 25th AUGUST 2001

What did I do today? Since I am writing this on Sunday night (tomorrow!!) I am looking back on today!? Oh yes, took J to my mum n dads and he stayed there, R came home. I was (am?) going out for a meal with Nicola, we were going to the nearby Indian but it was closed for refurbishments. So we went to a pub had a meal (Tai curry then a large Knickerbocker Glory!) and lager!! Then onto another pub with more lager!! Well, it was my belated birthday meal (another one!). Had fun looking round the pub at various blokes, unfortunately they were mostly ermmm... non-fanciable!

SUNDAY 26th AUGUST 2001

Went to my mum n dads to get J, but he wanted to stay another night and R decided to stay too (her first ever night away from home without me or N)! I kept ringing my mum all night to see if she was ok, but at least she is with her big brother. SO... well... N suggested we go out to eat (no need for babysitters), so we did. To an Italian restaurant, lovely. I had pasta n meatballs (called something Italian but it was pasta n meatballs) and a YUMMY dessert of cappuccino mousse.

I just can't get any of my clothes on... I've got to do something!!!! I've got to lose weight. NOW - NO MORE EATING OUT, AT ALL, FOR AGES, OK!!!!

Tomorrow is Monday and a NEW start, no waiting till the day after, the day after, the day after... next week, soon, when the kids go back to school, when I'm in the mood!!, when I've got more time to myself, when none of my clothes fit, when it's not period time, when I go healthy shopping, n all that. What was I saying?? Yes, tomorrow I will (yet again) start again.

New Week 1

Monday 27th Aug 2001

This is a new beginning and where I START to lose weight! Today...well...ok so I didn't eat too well, but it is (was) bank holiday, sunny and we went out and had brekky minus the kids!! I have decided (yet again!) to get counting points in an effort to control what I am eating. As I said before, Judith is gonna start coming round once a week again for us both to get weighed (and pay £1 plus an extra £1 for every lb we put on - that'll teach us!!) I will also begin to do some exercise (and got the ab-cruncher out at night!) and when R n J go to school I will get back to the gym (since I am paying for it each month) So, it's the gym on Mondays and Fridays and the odd Wed thrown in!

```
              Brekky - 2 toast
Lunch - All day brekky in OK Diner + pancakes
               n icecream.
       Tea - Iced Mocha in McDonalds
```

TUESDAY 28th AUGUST 2001

Today I count points (even with a cinema visit and a call in at MacDonald's, yes I know, another one, but J wants to go as it is part of the day out!)

WEDNESDAY 29th AUGUST 2001

Such a busy day! We went swimming, to the park, to a carboot sale, then an attic sale, then home (I am knackered!) Judith and I have been talking about how we are going to have to do it properly (THIS DIETING), no messing, or we will just not lose weight. Not long now before the kids go back to school (next week). NO MORE MCDONALDS!

```
                FOOD
    Brekky-cereal + skim milk
        Lunch-Ham sand
 Tea-Pepper chicken + piece pizza
```

Eve-Cereal + smilk

SATURDAY 1st SEPTEMBER 2001

Went to Llandudno today. Yesterday we went to Gulliver's World. All these days out of course, mean, well, eating the sort of stuff you eat on days out!!! BUT, the time is ticking away, soon, when Tuesday comes (kids back at school), it's time to get serious.

> WEIGHT
> 29/8/01 11st 7 lbs

New Week 2

TUESDAY 4th SEPTEMBER 2001

YES!!!!! I actually got through a day without silly picking. I ate really well today, better than I have done for ages.

OK, so now JUDITH if you are reading this, tomorrow is the DAY, you WILL come round to my house and get weighed and we WILL start sticking to this diet/healthy eating plan. NO WAY are we going to be this weight for Christmas!!

```
FOOD
Bfast - 2 toast
Lch - 3 bread + ham
Tea - New potatoes + 2 low fat sausage + veg +
1 apple
Eve - 1 toast
```

WEDNESDAY 5th SEPTEMBER 2001

Judith came round and we weighed ourselves. I was 11 st 6 lbs and she weighed 14 st 11 lbs. We are both really determined to LOSE IT this time. N went to the shop on the way home from work and got 3 packets of pink n whites marshmallow wafers (6 per pack), I haven't had these for ages and I just LOVE them. So I worked my way through all but 2 of them (N ate those). STUPID THING TO DO!

```
FOOD
Bfast - 2 toast
Lch - Ham sandwich
Tea - Shepherds Pie
Eve - 16 (yes 16) pink n whites (wafers with
marshmallow in the middle), 2 small bread
rolls with meat + 1 pac lit crisps
```

WEIGHT TODAY
11 st 6 lbs
loss so far = 1 lb

THURSDAY 6th SEPTEMBER 2001

I am going to aim to do some exercises tonight (feel knackered at the moment, but...). Did a lot of walking round the shops today and to and from school (so am now doing a bit more!!) Nibbled on the kids meatballs, the Swedish ones (yummy!). Must stop this picking.

```
FOOD
Bfast - Branflakes + smilk
Lch - Ham baguette + some chips
Anoon - some of the kids meatballs!
Tea - salad, chicken, 1 slice wmeal bread +
diet yoghurt + 2 packs lite crisps (eve)
```

FRIDAY 7th SEPTEMBER 2001

Not too bad a day, though I did have a hypo not long after lunch so ate some chocolate fingers. Judith has been ringing up, she is doing well on her diet (and not having alcohol!! - so she says!!)

```
FOOD
Bfast - branflakes+smilk
Lch - Wmeal roll+chicken+2teasp lite mayo
Anoon - Banana+choc fingers
Tea - Veg stirfry with noodles
```

SATURDAY 8th SEPTEMBER

OK day. Though had a hypo again mid-afternoon so had extra cereal. I am determined this time to start eating healthier and get seeing some weightloss. Was looking at an old photo of N, he looked so THINNER and to think back then I thought he was big!! I am going to bed feeling pleased with myself! YIPPEE!

```
FOOD
Bfast - 2 toast
Lch - Spanish omelette, 1 banana, 1 diet
yoghurt
Anoon - 2 bowls cornflakes
```

```
Tea - Strawberries + lite mousse
     Snack - I bread roll
```

Not the most balanced of eating days, but good all the same!

N weighs 19st 11 lb

SUNDAY 9th SEPTEMBER

It's when you can't be bothered thinking about what you might eat that you go and end up eating crappy stuff. I made a cooked breakfast this morning (don't know why, just felt like it). We never have cooked breakfast 'cept if we go out for it!! I didn't go mad!!! Then I went out for the rest of the day to my friend's house and just had lots of coffees there and eventually got home 6.30pm (having had nothing to eat all day) - clever of me!! So I did not eat too well when I got home, what a surprise!

```
                    FOOD
Bfast - 2 rashers bacon, 1 egg, 1 low fat
        sausage and 2 slices toast.
Tea - Pasta with tinned tomatoes with garlic.
Then I ate about 3/4 of a garlic baguette (low
        fat version), I ate 1 pop tart
    Eve - Low fat strawberry mousse.
```

Must eat better tomorrow!!

New Week 3

TUESDAY SEPTEMBER 11th 2001

Thinking of all those involved in the awful events that took place in the US

WEDNESDAY 12th September 2001

Seems silly really to be going on about what I have and what I haven't eaten in light of what has happened. Everyone is so shocked and saddened by it all. I wish I could go there to help in some way. It is the worst thing that I have ever seen (in my lifetime).

WELL DONE

Judith has lost 4 lbs, unfortunately I gained one, I obviously didn't do as well as I thought I had.

THURSDAY 13th September 2001

My mum came down today, we did loads of tidying and finished off the painting in J's room, so that's my exercise for the day! I ate my tea early, I bet I will be hungry later on, but I will aim to only have a small snack. Meant to do some exercise but I am too tired, went to bed early, N brought me up a cup of tea and toast!!

```
                    FOOD
             Bfast - 2 toast
Lch - 1 w'meal roll + meat + 1 half a sandwich
            (my mum bought for me)
          Anoon - 1 Muller lite rice
           Tea - Spag bol (homemade)
                Eve - 2 toast
```

WEIGHT TODAY
11 st 7 lbs
gained 1 lb

FRIDAY 14th September 2001

I asked N to pick up some chocolate for the kids on his way home (R was screaming the place down cos she didn't want her nanna and granddad to go, also she was very tired after her half day in pre-school). I made a lovely stew for tea (ermm...fairly healthy, just a few dumplings in it!). Of course N came home with the BIGGEST bag of sweets you can get, chocolate mostly! So what have we all been nibbling all night?? No wonder I feel so YUCK now. Trouble is, if it's there I EAT IT, my willpower is mainly crap. Now, if he had got just one or 2 chocolate bars, just enough for one each for the kids, all well and good - but to get a HUGE one?**##%*^'@***

```
                    FOOD
       Bfast - Branflakes + smilk
           Lch - Egg sandwich
          Anoon - 1 banana
        Tea - Beef Stew + 2 dumplings
Eve - 1 bread roll + meat + various chocolate
```

JUDITH'S WEIGHT
14 st 7 lbs
lost 4 lbs

NOTE
Spoke to Judith on the phone today (Friday), she is in an EATING mood. She said she ate a pile of cheese last night but was good otherwise (which IS GOOD). So LISTEN Judith, don't worry too much about what you think you might eat, just aim to eat healthy wherever possible and keep the PICKING/OVEREATING to a minimum (HEY - I should take my own advice here!!!!)

SUNDAY 16th September

Got to eat better, got to exercise more (or some at least!), got to stop picking, got to drink more water - if I wanna lose any weight!! I WANT to LOSE WEIGHT SO MUCH, arrgggg!! I feel like screaming!! I truly, truly am SO fed up of being this weight, I hate the way I look, hate all my clothes, hate my huge stomach, hate...anyway, I'm just in one of those moods!

```
                    FOOD
```

```
        Bfast - 2 toast
  Lch - I roll + meat + some choccie fingers
  Anoon - 1 and 1/2 pancakes + few pieces of
                  swiss roll
Tea - chicken in gravy + new potatoes + veg +
                  diet yog
    Eve - Egg custard, 1 roll + salad
```

DON'T EAT ANYTHING ELSE - JUST GO TO BED!!!

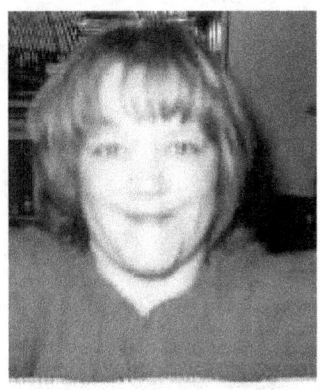

it's the body, it's HUGE!

New Week 4

TUESDAY 18th September

Today I am going to be good, I am not going to eat silly things. I was too tired to go on the exercise bike last night (N went on it though).

FOOD
Bfast - Branflakes +smilk + a banana

JUDITH'S WEIGHT
14 st 10lbs
GAIN 3 lbs

WEIGHT TODAY
11 st 8 lbs
GAIN 1 lb

WEDNESDAY 19th September 2001
WEIGHING DAY

Judith came round and we weighed ourselves.. How, HOW?? How do we put on weight so easily?? It is NOT FAIR, I never stuff myself (well, hardly ever)

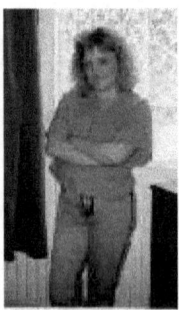

I want to be this slim again (NOW)

FRIDAY 21st September 2001

N has been on the exercise bike each night even though he has not been well. I just don't feel like I have the energy to do any exercise. Had to go to physio on my hand today (arthritis). I DO need to get back to the gym.

```
               FOOD
         Bfast - 2 toast
    Lch - ham n egg mayo baguette
       Anoon - 2 options drinks
         Tea - Noodles + veg
```

SUNDAY 23rd September 2001

Went to my mum's today, was ok. BUT, my sister came over and she kindly gave me her FAT clothes!! ARRGGG!!!!!!!!!! How could I have let it get to this?? This is just the worst thing ever. I mean, I am pleased that my sister has managed to lose 18 lbs, really I am. Couldn't be more pleased for her.

Rang Judith, she has been on a bit of an eating spree, ok so not as bad as me. When I was telling her the little extras I had eaten, the little extras added up to A MASSIVE AMOUNT. I have picked so much. God I feel depressed!

Me and Judith HAVE got to TRY HARDER - otherwise we'll be this weight at Christmas, next Summer, forever. Actually, being tall, Judith can get away with it much more than me (me being under 5ft), don't suppose there's any chance of me getting taller now??

New Week 5

MONDAY 24th September 2001

YEAH I went to the gym today. I haven't been there since June. I have now signed up for full membership, meaning I can go anytime and at weekends (N and the kids hate moving anywhere on a Sat morning and I am usually itching to get out of the house!)

```
              FOOD
        Bfast - 2 toast
    Lch - 2 wmeal bread, ham
       Anoon - 1 banana
 Tea - pasta, tomatoes. Diet yoghurt
     Eve - Rice-crispies
```

TUESDAY 25th September 2001

It's 8am, I am going to eat well today. N has gone off to work. Kids are about to get ready for sch. I have physio at 9.30am.

```
             FOOD
   Bfast - 2 bananas+apple
      Lch - Sandwich
  Anoon - can't remember
    Tea - Soup, 2 bread
 Eve - Chocolate, 2 toast
```

WEDNESDAY 26th Sept 2001

Well, Judith came round and we weighed ourselves. I am pleased to say I stayed the same. Judith was down about putting on 4 lb. We have to try harder (I keep saying this).

```
     FOOD - Dunno?
```

WEIGHT TODAY
11 st 8 lbs
Stayed the same

JUDITH'S WEIGHT

15 st

Gain of 4 lb

THURSDAY 27th Sept 2001

Been reading some slimming mags for inspiration and motivation (hasn't worked yet!)

SUNDAY 30th Sept 2001

I have been emailing Kathy in the US. We are Email Weightloss Buddies and we have been setting each other challenges each day, exercise challenges, just small ones to begin with. I feel it is SUCH a good idea and will help us get rid of this extra weight. THANKS KATHY!

Ok, ok, I admit it, I ate out today. Shouldn't have, but I did (N's fault!)

```
                    FOOD
 Brunch - meatballs n spaghetti. + chocolate
          dessert thing and 2 latte's.
 Tea - Steak and bread (couldn't be bothered
              with anything else)
```

Went to the gym on Friday, I stayed there an hour, I am glad I went even though I didn't get there till lunchtime!

New Week 6

MONDAY 1st October

Another week, I WILL do better!

```
               FOOD
Ermmm...what did I eat today??? Forgot to fill
it in! I think I did ok??? Even though we went
              shopping to Tesco!!
```

I will do it!!

TUESDAY 2nd Oct 2001

I have decided to do an exercise log!! I'm sure it all helps in the long run (and gives me something to do HA HA! Got an email from Kathy and she said another person is doing the exercise challenges (that is really great) and as she says "it is almost an exercise routine"! Keep this up and it will be our very own internet exercise class! Is it time to eat yet?? I am SO hungry, but I think it is mainly boredom. I have worked my way through half a pac of mini breadsticks and halfway round the web (along with cups of tea and coffee). Now all I want to do is eat. N is not due home till about 6pm/6.30 (it is now 4.30). When he gets home we can eat something tasty (but what do I do till then??) I am SO sick of drinking (not alcohol!, just tea n coffee and the ever so refreshing! green tea)

```
                 FOOD
          Bfast - 2 toast
   Lch - half ham baguette + lite mayo
      Anoon - some breadsticks
 Tea - Scrambled eggs and bacon, 2 small bread
      Eve - 2 bowls rice-crispies
```

Not a bad day eating wise! Though I think I will have to cut down the evening cereal to 1 bowl!!

Today I am going to be good and I am going to eat well and take to exercise.

Kathy is doing well and doing brilliantly with the exercise challenges that we set ourselves each day. She sets them one day, I set the next and so on. Judith has also joined in doing the challenges, she says she has to get her tins out!!! So, JUDITH, get the tins of beans out NOW.

WEDNESDAY 3rd Oct

WEIGHING DAY! I am just waiting for Judith to come round to get weighed, I wish she would hurry up (I want a cup of tea and of course if I drink it before I get weighed, well, I will weigh more!)

YIPPEE! I lost 1 lb and Judith lost 2 lbs - here we go!!!!

GOD what happened in the evening? I just pigged out, stupid or what? I did some exercise in the evening at least.

```
                    FOOD
              Bfast - 2 toast
      Lch - 1 toast, soup, 1 options drink
            Anoon - rich tea biccies
        Tea - Swedish meatballs, 1 bread
    Eve - erm....3 mini (very mini) cakes, 2
  choccie biscuits, small tub icecream, almost
            whole pac poppets (mint)
```

WEIGHT TODAY
11 st 7 lbs (161 lbs)
LOST 1 lb

JUDITH'S WEIGHT
14 st 12 lbs (208 lbs)
LOST 2 lb

Thursday 4th Oct

I....today I try harder! I blame my friend Kim, she bought me a HUGE box of biscuits from Cadburys factory, ok... I might have asked her to since they were so cheap. I only ate 6 in all, then I gave the box to N's mum and dad, aren't I good!

```
            FOOD
        Bfast -2 toast
     Lunch - Ham sandwich
Anoon, 6 biscuits, 2 options drinks
      Tea - pasta + chicken
  Eve - 2 toast, 5 rice-tea biscuits
```

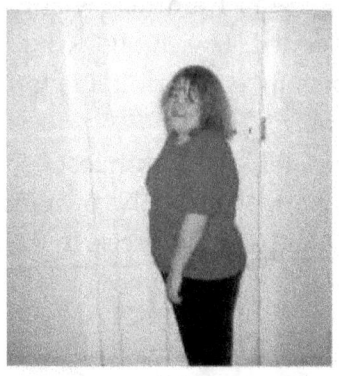

Just to remind myself why it is NOT GOOD
to eat chocolate biscuits

FRIDAY 5th Oct

Didn't do my challenges yesterday, felt ill (and no it was not the choc biscuits!). I might go to the gym today, dunno.

Well, I went to the gym, for an hour, now I am totally knackered!

```
            FOOD
   Bfast - 2 toast and a banana
Lunch - Jacket potato, chicken curry
```

At the gym I went on the treadmill 15 minutes, then the weight-machines which are air compressed, (makes them, easier for women!), then on the cross-trainer for 20 mins but actually only did 8 minutes. Drank plenty of water, sometimes

I forget and go on the stretching machine after having a drink of water then I feel REALLY PUKEY!

SATURDAY 6th Oct

Went to McDonalds (for the kids to have a play in the play tubes!) I had a Big Mac+Fries, but kept away from the ice-cream (which is good for me, I love their ice-cream). If I'm not careful between now and when I get weighed next I will definitely have put on weight.

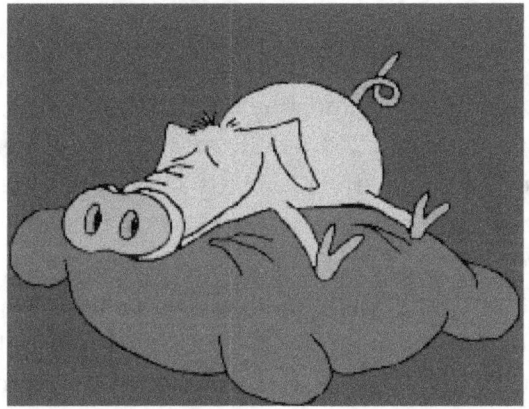

This is just how I have been feeling lately!

New Week 7

Monday 8th October

Went to the gym again today. Was v tired but made the effort. Now at the end of the day I have SO many aches!

Tuesday 9th October 2001

Last night....I don't even want to think about it. I can't believe what I did...well..I can...but. N went out shopping (I was too tired to go, so me and R stayed in). I said I felt like a LITTLE treat (well... I was aching and felt off colour). Anyway, N and J came home off Tesco with ...besides the bread we needed...2 LARGE packets of sweets. Namely Malteasers and Minstrels (just my fave!) I'm ashamed to say I must have had over half a bag of each and surprisingly I didn't feel too sick last night??

This morning (Tue)..ok I feel a little sick.

Cinnamon is quite good on a ham n tomato sandwich, you can hardly taste it. I am being v. lazy and just sitting around and reading. R is watching TV.

Been looking through the slimming world magazine and have a pile of ww ones nearby too....ohhhh and it's only 9.15 in the morning too!!! After last night....I feel I need to DO SOMETHING.

```
Bfast - branflakes+skim milk+2wwbread (as
          cinnamon toast*see note)
  Lunch - 4 ww bread+ham+tomato with a
          sprinkling of cinnamon
          Anoon - mini breadsticks
  Tea - spaghetti bol (homemade) and a banana
      Eve - bowl of rice crispies+smilk
```

* So you read these things...! I read that having a teaspoon of cinnamon with each meal was good...good if you have PCOS. And I think I might have it...seriously! So my inability to lose weight might be partly caused by PCOS (polycystic ovary syndrome)..which I was diagnosed with some yrs ago (when trying to get preg. with R). And if I don't have PCOS at all in any way shape or form, then cinnamon is hardly going to do me any damage (cept I will get sick of it!)

Wednesday 10th Oct

WEIGHING DAY (*groan*), the groan is because I have eaten so badly the last week.

YES! YES! YES!

I stayed the same weight, I am so pleased! And Judith lost a pounds, well done! Brilliant!

'Sfunny N never noticed the cinnamon in his Spag Bol last night!!

```
              FOOD
     Bfast - Branflakes + smilk
Lunch - ham n tomatoes sandwich (with added
              cinnamon!)
```

WEIGHT TODAY
11 st 7 lbs (161 lbs)
Stayed same

JUDITH'S WEIGHT
14 st 11 lbs (208 lbs)
LOST 2 lb

Thursday 11th Oct

S is exercise isn't it!! Right, ok. Today I am going to do more, exercise, well...I'll move about the house more!! HA, ha. My family are coming round tomorrow cos it is R's 4th bday and I JUST have to blitz the house before they get here - this is mega exercise!! Have decided not to bother writing down what I am eating since I rarely put down the whole days eating!?!. But I will probably have cinnamon toast for breakfast this morning!

'Sfunny how thinking about some people makes you want to lose weight (more so if you fancy them)...I know...I know I'm married. Mmmm.......where was I?

Friday 12th October

R's 4th birthday!! Party in McDonalds tonight (No I won't have a big mac!)

AND I didn't have the Big Mac (anyway they are yuck!)

Kids, more kids, noise, games, food, more kids, happy McDonalds people.......I AM TOTALLY KNACKERED! (can't think of a better way of putting it?). I sorta ate today, somewhere along the way. Haven't had much cinnamon lately!!

Sunday 14th October

Been a busy weekend! I have done very little in the way of exercise this week and I have done few if any of the challenges, I must get back to doing these (OK, Kathy - will do better this next week)

New Week 8

Monday 15th October 2001

Today I went to the gym for an hour, which I am really pleased about. I have had today's challenges from Kathy and so I am aiming to do them later tonight (hopefully). I must admit I am not looking forward to getting weighed on Wednesday. I am fed up of not getting anywhere FAST!!

Wednesday 17th October 2001 WEIGHING DAY!
(11st 7 lbs = 161 lbs - stayed the same)

JUDITH (15 st = 212 lbs - 4 lb gain)

YEAH, I stayed the same. Ok, so I am a teensy bit fed up of staying the same, a lot fed up actually. But, LOOK, if I actually made an effort and ate better then I WOULD actually lose weight!! N was upstairs when Judith stood on the scales downstairs (he heard the scream!)

Thursday 18th October 2001

N is off work with a bad stomach. I have eaten healthier today, apart from a few too many pieces of toast tonight.. I did some exercise tonight, I always leave it till too late and doing 40 side-bends and 40 leg raises + squats at 11pm at night is....well....not exactly the best time.

Friday 19th October 2001

We did some shopping today. And yes, I had some cream cakes (mini..well small ones and only..well only 3 (not too bad for me). Ok so I did eat some Stilton cheese with apricots in it, but I'd cut it in half and gave half away to a friend. I only had 2 ice-creams at night (while watching a video), oh yeah, and I just had 1 or maybe 2 packets of hula hoops sometime during the day. OK, OK, it was a ...crappy day eating wise, I didn't do so good. This can be my 1 day of overeating. THERE, it's DONE now, gone, I've eaten the stuff and now it's almost midnight. I feel a bit yucky really, suppose it's only to be expected?! AND guess what??? I just did 60 ab-crunches and 30 arm reaches..good aren't I!! Dunno HOW I did them, just did, guilt I think?!

Saturday 20th October 2001

I have healthy food in, no excuse not to eat better today. Dunno if I like the way this page is looking?? Did ok with the eating today in that I didn't overeat! Took the kids to Wacky Warehouse and we had something to eat afterwards, I had Lasagne (which was unfortunately very greasy) along with half a ciabatti bread and I skipped dessert, though I had a few spoonfuls of R's ice-cream! Had tea very late, 10.30, I had veg stir fry and pasta. Didn't do any exercise today.

Sunday 21st October 2001

J is sleeping at his cousin's. We have a film to watch tonight it's called *Shriek If You Know What You Did Last Halloween*! I am gonna try and do some exercise later (I hope!!)

New Week 9

MONDAY 22nd October 2001

Another new week, where I WILL do better. As I see it...I am taking Zotrim, cinnamon, exercising, drinking more water.. now the only thing I have to work on is the EATING!

My sister came down today, she looks great, so much thinner, I am so jealous (green!) I am going to DO it!! I did make chilli for my eve meal but ate it at 4pm cos I was so hungry. I only had the chilli, nothing else!!

TUESDAY 23rd October 2001

Went shopping for some Halloween stuff, guess where the kids are going for a Halloween party! Yep McDonalds, and I'm not even a big fan of the place but they do do a nice party (we went last year). While I was trooping round the shops, (with Judith + her kids + J), of course they got hungry and demanded food. We went into Sayers bakers, I had a coffee (although I was starving). The kids ate. On the way out, Judith said she didn't want me going hypo on her (true) and she bought me a pastie. We ate this back at my house, it was YUMMY but greasy. N is working late. I am going to try my best to do some exercise tonight (the ab-crunch/side-bends/bike sort!). It has got to help in the long run hasn't it???? We are out of photos on the instant Polaroid (N has wasted a few on candid ones of me AND I mean wasted! honestly, he ought to wait till I am at least 2 stone down- it's enough to put me off my food for life!)

I have not been able to go to the gym this week cos the kids are off school. R starts full-time pre-school next week, well, full time as in 5 mornings a week. I am still going to go to the gym Mon and Fri's and the odd other inbetween!!

WEDNESDAY 24th October 2001 (WEIGHING DAY)

YES! YES! YES! I went and lost a lb. I stepped on and off the scales 3 times to make sure. Just think how I could do if I REALLY tried! Not sure if Judith is coming round to day or not (with the kids being off school)? I have no plans for the day so far, except to keep sane and smile when the kids fight! I have decided to do a food log (and am going to count points in am attempt to... well... control what I am eating and eat better therefore to lose weight! That's the idea anyway!!

Weight Today
11 st 6 lbs (160 lbs)
Loss = 1 lb

THURSDAY 25th October 2001

Well, I started counting the points today. But N and I went out in the evening for our late anniversary meal. I really enjoyed it. So had far too many points yesterday, but still. I will do better today!

FRIDAY 26th October 2001

Didn't do too bad yesterday. It's the weekend and there's always a temptation to get a takeaway!!! Chinese!!?? Been having problems with getting the site updated it's a pain. There's been (there are) so many problems updating this site, it's really getting on my nerves (but haven't headed for the kitchen yet!)

SATURDAY 27th October 2001

Didn't really intend to, but we went out to eat (for the kids!). Little Chef (Boring!). Anyway, of course I had to eat (well, everyone else was). The kids enjoyed it cos they were giving away Rugrats toys with the meal. I had some light red wine in the evening. And serves me right, I came out in hives (heatlumps). I forgot I can't drink red wine, even the light stuff. God it's so bloody itchy.

SUNDAY 28th October 2001

So here we are at the end of another week. N weighed himself this morning, he has lost another lb, now he weighs 19 5. I am still suffering from the hives of last night (scratch, itch). Today...well...eating.....ate the wrongs things didn't I. We had Sunday dinner out, which was very nice, but did I have to have the dessert?? NO. But I did. We had a takeaway in the evening, did I have to have one too, NO. But I did. Mind you, it is next to impossible to watch all the family tucking into a takeaway and you have something different (however nice). Saw a good programme (with Alan Alda) on Obesity in America, it was called Fat and Happy. It was very good and funny. The conclusion (or one of them) it came to is that slow weightloss is best and that we most definitely need to eat fewer calories, plus it helps you live longer.

New Week 10

MONDAY 29th October 2001

Well, here I am in week 10. My weightloss so far (since the beginning of week 1) is a grand total of 1 lb. How do I do it!! This is not doing anything for my morale, motivation, mood, etc. BUT I am NOT going to give up. I think if I don't get losing some weight soon then people visiting this site will get fed up (?). It'll end up just being a diary not a weightloss site and I don't want this.

I didn't go to the gym today. Went to Kim's for a coffee and she was going to Tesco, so I went there instead.

WEDNESDAY 31st October 2001

Spooky...I lost another lb this week. I really don't know how? I weighed myself this morning, with my clothes on (all of them) and it said 11 5, I re-weighed myself 2 more times and it said 11 5. N was there as my witness! As you know I normally weigh myself later on in the morning when Judith comes to get weighed too (but I half guessed she wouldn't be popping round). I ate my brekky, had 3 glasses of water and a cup of coffee. Walked the kids to school, came home and thought I'd check my weight again (yeah, like it changes!). Oh and it did. The scale said 11 8, I dived off, on again at 11 9, off, on again at 11 7. Didn't do a lot for my motivation, but HEY I will go with the 11 5 cos it said it 3, yes 3 times.

We are going to McDonalds tonight for the Halloween party. The kids are eating I'm aiming not to!!

TODAY'S WEIGHT
11 stone 5 lbs
(159 lbs)
Loss 1 lb

THURSDAY 1 November 2001

I was SO good in McDonalds last night. I only had 1 plain burger, lots of coffees and ok so I had a few spoonfuls of J's ice-cream sundae, only a few!! It was good. J won a prize, he was dressed as Harry Potter, he looked wonderful. AS you can see from the photo, here is our very own Harry Potter (photo taken by McDonalds)

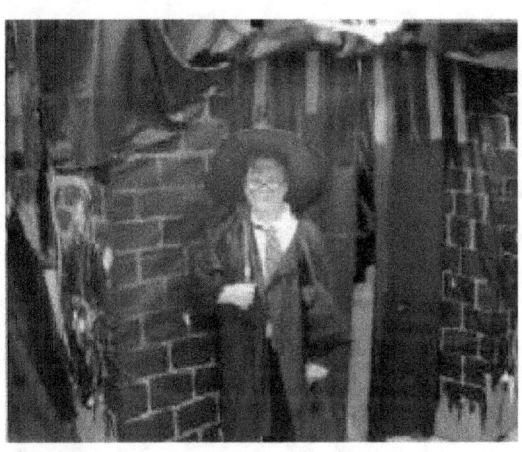

FRIDAY 2nd November 2001

Went to the hospital this morning for another check on my breast lump (I have had 2 other checks). The consultant said the lump was clear but did I want it removed (to stop me worrying), I said yes. I thought maybe they could do some liposuction while they are at it (I wish!) Went to my sister-in-law's in the evening, her son's birthday party (with fire-works). I ate far too much.

SATURDAY 3rd November 2001

Went to the supermarket and got some fruit, veggies etc but then proceeded to eat crappily the rest of the day (sweets and chocolate attack), now I feel sick, quite sick. I have got to try harder. Kathy in Ohio, my dieting friend is doing well with her weightloss and is still doing the exercise, which I am failing to do at the moment. She is sending me her daily food log, I am supposed to do mine but keep conveniently forgetting. I have to try to do better or I will not want to get on the scales on Wednesday.

WEEK 1 of Slimming World

MONDAY 5th November 2001

1st weigh-in: 11 stone 12 lbs (166 lbs)

Now this is gonna confuse people totally! Tonight I joined Slimming World. I was driven to it by my body (of all things!!). I am so fed up. I need to go along to something each week and, well...be motivated. Don't get me wrong, I have Kathy in Ohio and Judith, both of whom are helping me, we are helping each other (I hope). But I need some more help. And, ok, it's gonna cost me £3.25 a week, plus it gets me out of the house, it's very social. All I can say is it's worth a go. So here we are. I went along tonight, after having a HUGE meal, well, hugeish. My bladder was full, my belly was full, all my clothes on!! So, <u>no</u> comment about my starting weight, from here-on it's downwards!!

TUESDAY 6th November 2001

YES! YES! YES! I have gotten through a day not picking. Ok so it's 8.30 in the evening and there's a little way to go yet, but I know at the end of this day I will have done well. I have followed the slimming world programme (perhaps it was easier cos I had an <u>un-hungry day</u>!!??) Who knows, whatever, I am pleased with myself. I feel more determined this time. I know I can do it, I know I can eat sensibly and lose this extra weight.

WEDNESDAY 7th November 2001

I have been eating ok today too! Hypos might be a bit of a problem, but once I get my blood sugars sorted out, then it will be fine.

FRIDAY 9th November 2001

I have had a date to go in for my breast lump removal, 12th December. I expect to be in just 2 or 3 days.

I have stuck to this slimming world programme so well since I started it on Tuesday. It takes a little getting used to. Mainly I have stopped picking (must've caught me on a good week!!). Hopefully I will be able to keep it up and lose this weight. Really I think it was time to try another slimming club, I don't think it would matter too much which one. At this moment I need all the inspiration and motivation and support I can get. And I can get it at Slimming World, our consultant is called Leah.

SATURDAY 10th November 2001

I am being good still and have not felt terribly hungry so far. I am quite looking forward to going to Slimming World on Monday night.

SUNDAY 11th November

Went to my mum's for the day. Nessa has lost 1 st 9 lbs (I saw her card!!) I have been sticking to the plan all week. Even when we went to the cinema last night I was good. We went to see Harry Potter, it was very good and we really enjoyed it.

Week 2 of Slimming World

MONDAY 12th November 2001

> 2nd weigh-in: 11 st 11 lbs
> 1 lb loss so far

Get weighed today, I think I am looking forward to it!!??_I think I may have lost about 2 lb (I wish it were more), but, whatever, I will be glad of any loss!! Went to the diabetic clinic today saw Dr Jones (whenever I see him I always think of the Aqua song Dr Jones, Jones....calling Dr Jones...), he is so suntanned and white teeth and everyone fancies him (my Dr at the clinic that is)! Hehe!!!!! Anyway, I must try harder with SWorld, to lose this weight and improve my blood sugars. Well, I went to the meeting and I lost 1 lb. I am a little disappointed I must admit, but I am even more determined to stick to it. Actually if I lost 1 lb each week and kept doing so, well, eventually I'd be my ideal weight wouldn't I. So, onwards and....whatever, I will do it.

WEDNESDAY 14th November 2001

I have put a new page online, a page of photos of me when I was thinner (just to prove I once was!). If I was brave i would put up my most fat photos, but as yet I am not that brave!! Today I did not feel well, all achy and fluey, felt like crap really and was walking round like an old woman (looked a bit like one too). The kids are off school sick too (but back in tomorrow I hope). Today cos I felt ill, funnily enough I felt like the biggest bar of chocolate you can imagine, what I mean is, I felt like eating the biggest bar of chocolate (or biggest box of chocolates) you can buy. Luckily for me N would not go get me any (I feel so sorry for myself)! This is one time where comfort food would have been really justified, honest.

FRIDAY 16th November 2002

I so wanted to eat anything at all today, without thinking, without worrying whether I could/should or not. It must be SO nice to not have to worry about what you eat.

SATURDAY 17th November 2001

Dunno how the weekend is going to go??

I cannot sleep, it is late, well actually it is 4.45 Sunday morning and everyone is fast asleep. If I wasn't so lazy I would go make myself a drink, but.......ermmm to be truthful, it's too spooky to go downstairs (maybe I watch too many horror films?) I could just do with a hot chocolate drink and maybe a piece of toast (after all it is almost breakfast time!!)

SUNDAY 18th November 2001

This is the worst day of eating I have had for some time. We went out for the day, I did well here and was not tempted. Ate in a cafe and I just had a bowl of tomato soup and a roll. Because it was late when we got home we ordered Chinese - now here goes.......I had spring rolls, beef in bb sauce, prawn crackers and to top it all off I had a bag of malteasers and half a mars bar!

I am so annoyed with myself but I will go on and do better!

Week 3 of Slimming World

MONDAY 19th November 2001

> 3rd weigh-in: 11 st 8 lbs
> Loss = 3 lbs
> Total loss so far 4 lbs

Well, this is my Slimming World weigh-in day. I have no idea how I have done, but fingers crossed.

YES! I went to my slimming club and hopped on the scales and I have lost 3 lbs! I got off them quick in case they changed their mind! I am SO pleased and this will definitely motivate me for the rest of the week. AND I got my ball on the tree!!

TUESDAY 20th November 2001

Only plans for today are to go round to my friends for coffee and chat about next yrs hols and I will take my lunch there (cottage cheese and jacket potato + some for her, she's vegetarian)

WEDNESDAY 21st November 2001

Diana in New Jersey asks me what are cream teas, these are usually a cup of tea, a scone with fresh cream (thick) with strawberry jam (what you call jelly I think). Malteasers are small chocolate covered malty balls, honeycomb, crispy - I love them and Weetabix is a breakfast cereal, square wheat things that go mushy when you add hot milk. NOW I am hungry, I wasn't before!

I have eaten well today, as in, not too much! I run a mail order catalogue and they occasionally send you a small gift as a reward for being a good customer/agent (mostly something naff), well they sent a gift the other day, nice it was. They sent a box of Belgium chocolates, not just a small box but a 2 layered box. The kids and N saw it and insisted that I open it

(I just didn't want to). BUT I did! For the kids of course. Lovely centres, orange truffle, praline, rum, cappuccino, marzipan etc. Not the sort of centres the kids like unfortunately. R bit into a few, it was such a shame to waste them, so I didn't. I didn't eat many, just 4......to begin with, ermm.... I believe I had 6, 7 ok maybe 8 after that. It is so naughty of the kids not to eat them all and N only had a few despite me trying to force them on him. Anyway, they are gone now.

SATURDAY 24th November 2001

Mother-in-law's birthday, I did my best at the buffet! I also had a meal out last night and I was the only one who didn't have dessert! Ok, so we had a take-away the night before that (again I didn't eat too much). All in all though I don't expect any weight-loss this Monday, I will be keeping my fingers crossed for staying the same. I shall of course wear my lightest clothes, wear my contact lenses instead of glasses and summer sandals or slippers, or even take my shoes off before I stand on the scales. AND nothing shall cross my lips several hours before. Why OH Why do we do this!!!

Week 4 of Slimming World

MONDAY 26th November (Slimming World Weigh-in Day)

11 st 7

LOSS = 1 lb

<u>Loss so far = 5 lbs</u>

I really don't know what the scales will say tonight, I do feel I have 'picked' more this last week. I hope I have either stayed the same or lost a teeny bit??

WOW! I lost weight again, I am really pleased to say. I must keep this up. Spoke to my sister on the phone, she is flagging a bit, she's been doing SWorld since last May (she admits she's getting fed up). She has done SO well, I hope she keeps at it.

TUESDAY 27th November 2001

I feel so motivated after last night (the weigh-in). It also helps I am not that hungry cos I have a blocked nose!! I was in my friends house yesterday (she is tall and slim), she was trying clothes on for Christmas parties (boo hoo, I never get to go to any). I caught sight of myself in her wardrobe mirror and (can I swear here????) I looked BLOODY awful, really and truly awful. Ok, so I am not going to grow in height, I will never ever be tall, I can accept this. But do I have to be so WIDE and ROUND?? I keep picturing myself, how I looked and I cannot get it out of my mind (it's like a nightmare!). <u>I am going to avoid mirrors for the time being.</u>

WEDNESDAY 28th November 2001

Judith came round this morning to get weighed, she is 15 st 1 lbs (sorry for putting this online Judith!) I have been eating ok today! I should get going doing some exercises (regularly), me and Kathy are doing the challenges again, nothing too complicated to begin with. Just something we can do during the day (when we have a spare 5 minutes).

SATURDAY 1st December 2001

Went to see Jack n The Beanstalk today, it was nice, I ate just a few sweeties! How have I been with my eating...well, not too bad I suppose.

Week 5 of Slimming World

MONDAY 3rd December 2001

> 11 st 3 lbs
> Loss = 4 lbs
> Loss so far = 9 lbs

Another weigh-in day (or rather night). After the weigh-in tonight we all go to the pub for the slimming club's Christmas Meal. I am very much hoping that I lose at least 1 lb tonight, I'll be even more pleased with 2 lb!

OH WOW. I cannot believe it, I went to the slimming club tonight and got weighed, I lost 4 lb this week, making 9 lbs so far. I was so shocked and I stayed on the scales just looking at them (the women weighing me said "you can get off now"!) After we all got weighed we went to the pub for our Christmas Meal (it was nice) and I didn't go mad!!!

TUESDAY 4th December 2001

A good day, I am still feeling fantastic cos of the weigh-in last night. Ok, so I am only human and I did have a few chocolates that I have set aside for Christmas, it is almost Christmas.

FRIDAY 7th December 2001

I have hardly written anything lately. I have been nibbling, naughty me!! I am torn between buying in lots of goodies in preparation for Christmas and ermmm...not doing so. Of course I will have to get things in for the kids and well, to be honest we don't get many visitors (we do the visiting, much to N's dismay!). I guess I ought to have a balance of stuff in, healthy stuff and stuff the kids will like with a few nice extras thrown in!

Well, it is getting late and I am going to have a low fat yoghurt in a while, because I feel like one (good enough reason!). I always used to think of Friday nights as the time to 'pig out', ok so, I kinda did it lots of other nights too, but, Fridays are THE night to treat and indulge yourself, aren't they??!

Saturday 8th December 2001

Ate well today. I took R to a party and there was lots of food on offer and I didn't even have a nibble. I do keep worrying about putting weight on on my next weigh-in. I should say to myself "so what if I do, it's not the end of the world".

Been feeling down the last day or so, don't know why really, well, I do really, it's a number of things - all silly, but there you go.

Sunday 9th December 2001

R has another party to go to today, more tempting nibbles on offer, but I shall decline!! I am more determined than ever to lose this weight, so I'll go with it while I can!

Week 6 of Slimming World

Monday 10th December 2001

> 11st 2 lbs (156 lbs)
> Loss 1 lb
> <u>Loss so far = 10 lbs</u>

Well another day of getting weighed. PLEASE, PLEASE, PLEASE let me have lost some more weight!! People say that when you lose 10 lbs you go down a dress size?? Well, I sort of have (depends on the make!)

Well I lost another pound, This is brilliant. I actually got into a skirt that has been too small. I tried it on this afternoon. I haven't eaten well today, as in, I have only eaten some cereal for breakfast and a banana not long ago (it's 9.30pm). I just had no appetite today. I must make sure I eat properly (ha, what a thing for me to say!!) When I am in the hospital, well, they never give you too much food do they!!

Wednesday 12th December

Today I go into hospital to have my breast lump removed,(they are doing the op Thursday morning)so I won't be doing any entries for the rest of the week (I expect to be out of hospital Friday or Saturday at the latest (I stay in hosp. longer because I am diabetic)

Friday 14th December (home again)

Came out of hospital today. The op went well. My r-breast is sore but ok, I have staples in it which I get removed next week. Then I have to go back to the breast clinic in 4 weeks for a check-up. It is nice to be home, if tiring!! I have to be careful not to lift/move stuff etc for the next 4 to 6 weeks (hehe no housework or shopping!!)

Week 7 of Slimming World

Monday 17 December 2001

> WEIGHT = 11st 1 (155lbs)
> Loss = 1 lb
> Total loss so far
> 11 lbs

I cannot believe Christmas is coming up SO fast! WEIGH-IN tonight!! I am sort of looking forward to getting weighed, though I don't think I have eaten well this last 2 weeks. I did have a takeaway last night (just the meat dish nothing else...ohhhh...I did have a few spring rolls and a few prawn crackers EEEKKKK!! It was a nice treat! I thought to myself, what day am I on today (red or green, that's the slimming world plan) and luckily it was not an off day. I am dreading it when I get a HUGE 'gotta stuff my face with anything and everything' feeling. Crudities (little bits of raw carrot/lettuce/cucumber etc) just do not do. I am getting a digital camera (yippee), perhaps lots of gross photos of me all over the place will keep me in line!!!!!!

Tuesday 18th December 2001

YES! I lost yet another pound. I cannot believe how well I am doing. I won a bottle of diet coke too! 11 lbs, not many more and it's a whole stone gone.

Wednesday 19th December 2001

Went to pre-school today and saw R in her play, she was an elf. She looked beautiful, they all did. Yes there was a tear in the corner of my eye!

I do have to be careful, with more chocolate being around, it is so tempting to treat myself (too often).

I now have my digital camera, some piccies will shame me into not eating too much (this does not always work unfortunately).

Friday 21st December 2001

Been taking piccies with my new camera, still it is hard to get decent ones, perhaps when my double chins have gone!!???? I had my staples out today, it was not as painful as I imagined.

OK, OK... confession time. I have pigged out yesterday. I had nearly a whole box of matchmakers, then some choccie biccies, then some smarties THEN... ermmmm... it is easy to lose track you know!!! Kathy, if you read this PLEASE tell me off!!!!

Saturday 22nd December 2001

I have eaten a load of treacle toffee today (ugg, so high in fat and sugar), but it was so nice. I am not getting weighed this coming week, I next get weighed on 30th December. I DON'T want to have put loads on - this would make me SO sick. I keep deleting/erasing all the photos taken of me on the digital camera, I take one look at them and ohhhh.....I can't put that on line!!

Week 8 of Slimming World

Monday 24th December 2001

Well, here we are Christmas Eve. I am panicking a bit about all the bits and bobs I am eating. I daren't step on the scales. It seems silly to be saying "oh I will be good " in the middle of Christmas, when everyone has a great time eating and drinking what they want. I shall be sensible.

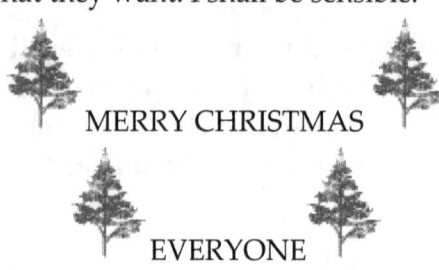

MERRY CHRISTMAS

EVERYONE

Thursday 27th December 2001

Well, We all had a lovely Christmas Day. And YES I did eat just what I wanted. I felt sick today though...I never want to eat any chocolate ever again! Trouble is, when the stuff is there in front of you (any stuff, whatever it is even if you are not keen on it!) you just well...eat it. especially when you go to other peoples houses, they have prepared it especially, so you gotta eat it. I am supposed to be getting weighed on Sunday night....I AM dreading it. BUT, not to worry.....I have been doing so well so far, Christmas is certainly not going to spoil my efforts (temporarily it will yes...but that is all!)

Christmas Photos

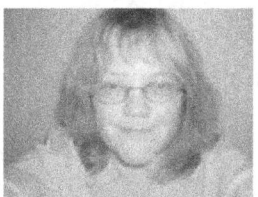

Here I am looking knackered!

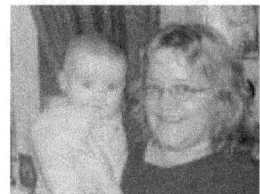

Me and my Niece Amie

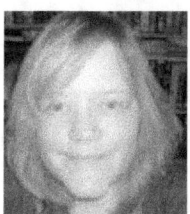

I avoid showing the rest of my body (hehe!)

Friday 28th December 2001

My 2 have been up all night (so have N and I), they, the kids were throwing up all night, there is a bug going round and my 2 have it. J is not at all well, they are both feeling so sicky.

Sunday 30th December 2001

N has got the sicky bug too, he was up all night puking etc. It's certainly a fast bug. So far obviously I have escaped it. I go get weighed tonight! It is very difficult to get back into eating sensibly after all the 'extra' eating. Luckily we don't have all the christmassy type stuff left in the house. The kids and us have worked our way through the chocolate and I avoided buying cakes n mince pies etc (aren't I good) - I just ate them at other peoples houses!!!!

Well I went and got weighed and I only put 1 lb on, just 1 lb, not bad for Christmas!! I am pleased. My aim now is to eat healthier, whilst I haven't gained much weight, it isn't because I have been eating healthy (I have eaten small amounts with picking chocolates).

> Slimming World Weigh-In
> Today's Weight = 11st 2 lbs (156 lbs)
> Gain 1 lb
> Total lost so far = 10 lbs

2002

Week 9 of Slimming World

Monday 31st Jan 2001

Today is normally weighing in day, but we got weighed yesterday - I had gained 1 lb, which is great considering the time of year!

Tuesday 1st Jan 2002

I was going to be so good today and I was almost. I ate a good breakfast and we went shopping, not for anything interesting, just for a piece of board for R's bed. They were with their nan and granddad so I thought we ought to get them a McDonalds. And because McDonalds food is not THAT filling, I over bought. So I got too much and of course the kids ate very little (just wanted the toy). So I ended up having 3 burgers and 1 portion chips-ok so not a mega pig out, but what a waste. I felt yuck after it, not particularly full or satisfied.

Wednesday 2nd Jan 2002

Oops, I pigged out last night, with the help of a bit of alcohol (ha blame that). So it was the McDonalds, tea was ok, then I had half a bottle of Martini (I did win it at a fair!) and it was opened and I didn't have any other alcohol all over Christmas (ok so I had a bit when I went to my mums - she offered! and at my sisters - they were all having a Christmassy drink so I didn't want to be a killjoy). So ermm, back to last night. Yep, I had the martini (very nice it was), then N was making hotdogs (which I don't like at all) but I had 2 of them.

Oh well, I suppose 2 hot dogs is not too much pigging out, I don't think I ate anything else???? No I didn't, I definitely didn't - so aren't I good. Feel better now!

Nessa (my sister) put 3 and a half pounds on over Xmas, she is off to her Slimming World meeting tonight.

I always want to eat when I feel stressed out and for various reasons I feel mega stressed out at the moment. Just as well there isn't anything too fattening in the house. Though I am off to my sister-in-law's soon (it is her birthday) and it is very tempting to see what goodies she has in to scoff.

I went to my sister-in-law's and I did have a few chocolates (about 8). N has just IM'd (instant messaged me) from work and asked are we having a takeaway? How could he! I can eat Chinese, on a red day, if I'm careful, if I be good the rest of the week, if I avoid spring rolls n prawn crackers, if I just stick to one dish, just boiled rice, no picking, no finishing off others, no tasting others - I know I can. I have been visiting the pages of other slimmers, I forgot how interesting it can be and how motivating it can be too.

Ermmm... we had that Chinese! Oh it was so tasty. What can I do to counteract the damage??? Exercise? Less food for the next ....?? I did have some spring rolls (just 4) and the rest (won't bore you with all I ate! It's N's fault, he made me). Now I am SOOOOO full up. R and J enjoyed it too.

Thursday 3rd Jan 2002

I went on the create your own virtual model site, it's ok, but I had to add at least 50 lbs to my model (on top of my actual weight) for her to look like me! The virtual models legs are MUCH fatter than mine. Actually my legs are sort of skinny which does not go with the rest of me at all - I just look stupid! If I had the money and was brave enough I would have the op that re-shapes your stomach, not that I am lazy and don't want to diet of course. Nessa lost 2 lb (well done!).

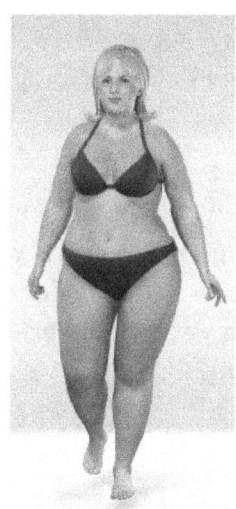

My virtual model.
My fat is not so evenly distributed unfortunately!

I have just started reading a book by Sherry Ashworth called Let's Get Physical. The blurb on the back says.....

Fit not Fat...words that strike terror into Cassies's ample bosom. But she has no choice; she loses either her excess weight or her gall bladder. With the scalpel of Damocles hanging over her, she joins the gym for the first time in her life, and learns that health is the new religion. Meanwhile Jane, the Manager at the Fit not Fat Healthclub has her work cut out....It's a race against time for Jane to prove herself and Cassie to lose those pounds. But is there a price to pay for the single minded pursuit of fitness? And why are we all so obsessed by health?

So far I am into the first chapter and I am really enjoying it, it is really funny. If you are interested you might find it at Amazon or somewhere like that. I was lucky and got it free with Slimming Magazine (UK, not sure if available in US)

Friday 4th Jan 2002

We went shopping and I got armed with healthy foods! I don't think I will have lost any weight this coming week since I HAVE been well....overeating. Silly me! The kids are stressing me out, it's too cold to eat healthy foods and I haven't got the energy to do anything - that about sums me up at the moment.

Saturday 5th Jan 2002

Why is it that when I go to my mums for the day...I always end up eating far too much?? I was gonna be so good n all. But, saying that, I have done exercise for the last 2 nights. I dusted off my trusty old exercise video and managed half of it last night and tonight.

Week 10 of Slimming World

Slimming World Weigh-In
Weight This Week = 11 st 1 lb (155 lbs)
Pounds lost = 1 lb
Total Lost So Far = 11 lb

Monday 7th January 2001

The kids go back to school today. I am really not sure how I will do tonight at the weigh-in. I was planning on going to the Gym today but can't go now for various reasons. I will try to go on Friday.

YES! I lost the lb I put on over Christmas!!!! I feel Sooooo good!!

Wednesday 9th January 2002

Am suffering with my arthritis at the moment (probably that exercise I did the other 2 nights!) So I'll give exercise a miss for a short time. Well, till next week anyway. I went to my slimming world meeting on Monday, and as everyone said, I just have to lose 3 more lb and I will have lost a stone. I was so motivated at the meeting but now I feel like it's something I have to do (lose 3 lb) and I know I won't do it.

Saturday 12th January 2002

Can't stop picking. A nibble here a nibble there. N got donuts and cakes tonight, it is Sooooo tempting and how HOW can anyone ignore the goodies?? I mean, even when you are not hungry you want to eat nice things don't you?! So, I know for definite that I will not have lost 3 lb this week, as it goes I will be lucky to have lost any. Bugger!!

Week 11 Of Slimming World

Slimming World Weigh-In
Weight this week = 11st (154 lbs)
Pounds lost = 1
Total lost so far = 12

Monday 14th January 2002

Get weighed tonight!! I am SO glad I joined Slimming World, I got weighed tonight and have lost another lb.

Tuesday 15th January 2002

I am so pleased that I lost another lb. I am going to France in July and I really would like to be my ideal weight then. It can be done, I CAN do it. I have to keep reminding myself, especially when I 'roam' the kitchen in search of food!!!!!

Thursday 17th January 2002

I have been trying stuff on from my wardrobe...of course the stuff doesn't fit (ha that would be silly!!) It acts as a motivator (when I am in good mood) and makes me feel SO down when I am not in a good mood!

Friday 18th January 2002

I went for a check at the breast clinic today (the lump removal was on 13th December). The consultant gave me the all clear and I don't have to go again!!! I wandered round the shops and popped into a hairdressers and had my hair done (I felt I needed some pampering!). I am reluctant to spend money on new clothes cos, well.....I don't intend to be this size for long (fingers crossed!) Ermmmm....okay so tonight I ALSO treated myself to a Chinese takeaway but I didn't overdo it!!

Saturday 19th January 2002

I am going to try and be good. I stood on my scales at home (shouldn't have) and I.. well.. I look like I weigh the same, but I want to weigh less. I want to be 10 stone something instead of 11. I don't feel I have tried very hard this week. Judith is doing the Atkins diet and is weighing herself at Boots the Chemist once a week. This 1st week she has lost 3 lb. Which is brilliant. She seems to be following the diet ok, I don't think I would have the will power to do it.

WELL DONE KATHY

Kathy, my friend in Ohio is regularly losing the weight. She is doing SO well, I know she gets fed up with her weight. She has a great sense of humour and is a wonderful diet buddy too (tells me off when I need it!).

Week 12 of Slimming World

Slimming World Weigh-In
Weight Today = 11st 1 lb (155 lbs)
Weight Gain = 1 lb
Total Lost So Far = 11 lbs

Monday 21st January 2002

Here we go again!! Another weighing day. I just know I have put weight on this week and I DON'T want to go and get weighed. Silly I know. I know I will feel down in the dumps if I have put even 1 lb on. I am almost in the mood to miss the meeting, but I know if I do then I can miss it again and again etc. I need to keep going and accept that some weeks I will put some weight on (being human n all). I feel I have eaten badly this last week. It's like a big black cloud hanging over me now. Wish I didn't feel like this. And truthfully I know how silly it is. As you can see I gained 1 lb. I felt SO depressed about it. I never stayed to the meeting, went shopping. Bought some biscuits. Got home ate about 10 biscuits (they were small, that is my only defence!), I also ate 2 large pieces of chocolate cake. STUPID. But I have gone and done it now. I have made a plan for tomorrow and I will eat healthily. I am over feeling down (sort of) and well, now I'll just get on with it again - get on with eating better to lose weight for next week.

Wednesday 23rd January 2002

I am TRYING to be good really I am. When you 'lose it' it's so easy to get back into picking. I got my exercise bike downstairs (nearly killed me carrying it, or rather plonking down each stair). It was in the bedroom holding clothes so I thought it was about time we used it.

Thursday 24th Jan 2002

I am reduced to eating dry cereal... not just any old cereal, but children's chocolate flavoured cereal. I never meant to eat it. R likes to have a bowl of it to munch on, as kids do. And without realising it I had nibbled my way through a bowl of it (her bowl, she complained and asked for more)! She said "Oh Mummy.....where's it all gone"? I looked and indeed it HAD all gone and we all know where (as I glance down at my stomach!)

Slimming World Week 13

Slimming World weight = 11 st. (154 lbs)
Loss = 1 lb Total Loss So Far = 12 lbs

Monday 28th January 2002

Well I lost the lb I put on last week, thank goodness!

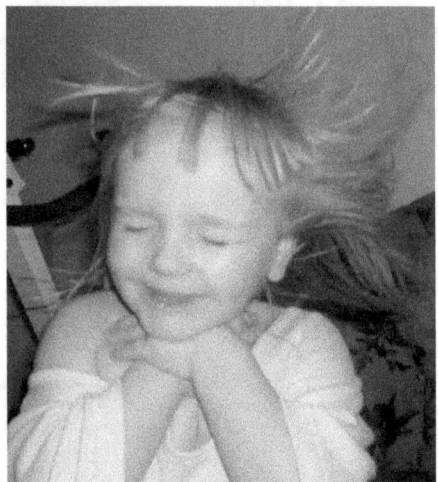

Here is my favourite little girl having her hair dried, this photo always makes me smile!

Thursday 31st January 2002

Well January has not actually been good for weightloss. I have not lost a lot. I have been a bit fed up really and I get annoyed with myself when I eat rubbishy things. My good intentions don't seem to last long, or rather, I let things get to me then I go eat all the stuff I have been avoiding in order to lose weight. I do not want to spend the whole of February juggling 1 lb off and on. Tomorrow night I am going to my friends house, she is having a late celebration, she was 40 a week or so ago. So, there will be about 9 of us there. We have bought Asda curry's between us, which happen to be free on the Slimming World plan, and a few of us are following it. Ok, so I shall have maybe just a few glasses of alcohol, but not too many!!!!!!!!!!!!!!!!!!

Friday 1st Feb 2002

Went to Kim's in the evening. I had some of the starters (samosa etc, mini ones), spring rolls, I nibbled the nuts! Then we ate the Indian dishes, all free on the Slimming World plan, I never had rice. Then I had a small piece of fruit flan. But there was a lovely strawberry sponge cream cake, no one, but no one had any. They all ignored it saying they were full. How could they?? I looked at if for ages. Then I thought, well, it's fresh cream and it can go off and Kim would be left with it. So I had a small piece. Wow it was nice, sort of light. So I had some more. Finally I looked at the cake again, a good 1/4 of it had gone. So I figured I had better stop. If I am honest, I could've eaten the whole thing!! Also I had a few after eight mints. Oh and one bottle of light wine.

It was a nice night!

Sat 2nd Feb 2002

Nessa came down. She lost 3 lb last week. We chatted about weight etc. I have bought various clothes ready for the hols in the summer, they fit me but only just! So Nessa tried them on, they looked fine on her (I was a bit jealous!) She wants to lose about 10 more lbs. I WANT to be thinner, please, please, please!! I felt more motivated. I had decided not to go to Slimming World on Mon night but hah, Leah phoned (the SW consultant). I am SO glad she phoned, cos now I AM going to the meeting Mon night.

OH, we went out for a meal in the evening, me N and J. J has just taken his 11+ so this was a treat for him. We told R we were going shoe shopping (she hates this), N's mum and dad babysat R. For the meal I was pretty good. Soup, steak, new potatoes, veg then an ice-cream bomb (should've had fruit salad!!!).

I wish I could enjoy trying clothes on.

Sunday 3rd feb 2002

I feel SO fat, I am sure I have put loads on, really I have. Why did I eat so much this last week?? Can't turn the clock back.

Slimming World Week 14

Slimming World Weigh-In
Weight = 10 st 13 lbs (153 lbs)
Loss = 1 lb
Total loss So Far = 13 lbs

Monday 4th Feb 2002

YES! I lost another lb. Ok, so after the meeting I treated myself to a piece or 3 of chocolate cake-but...but that's all I will do. Oh, yeah, I did have just one small danish. OK, big treat done, gone, out of the way. I shall be good all week.

Thursday 7th Feb 2002

Had a lazy day today really. Went on the scales and they read much lower!!!! So what did I do late afternoon??? I ate some chocolate biscuits of course. Why oh why do I do it?? I have no excuse. I must try and go on the bike tonight, knackered knees or no knackered knees!

Sunday 10th Feb 2002

I have nibbled my way through the weekend. I have eaten things I didn't mean to, didn't intend to. Though saying that, I got a skirt out of my wardrobe that simply would not fasten on me, and now it does! YIPPEE!!

Slimming World Week 15

Slimming World Weigh-In
Tonight's Weight = 10st 12 lbs(152 lbs)
Loss = 1 lb
Total Loss So Far = 14 lbs

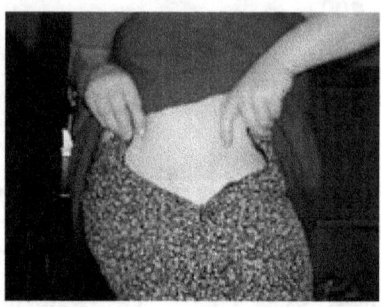

As you can see I have taken a photo of me in a skirt I truly want to get into and as you can see, I'm a long way off!!!!! I am really loath to say this but here goes...the left hand side of the photo is my stomach ARRGGGHHH!!!!! Mega gross or what! N says it's the weirdest photo he ever saw (he took it!!), I am twisting sideways. Bloody hell I look pregnant!

Monday 11th Feb 2002

I have no idea how I have done this last week. I admit I have popped on and off my scales and they have said 10st 10 lbs (which is 150 lbs). I have been nibbling on chocolate all week, because.. well.. it's been there. So it's no good me saying "please... please... please let me have lost loads of weight... at least 2 lb" is it??!!!!

OK, I lost 1 lb. I got a certificate for losing a stone and a snazzy sticker on my book! I must try harder. I am pleased with my weightloss so far, I am. But part of me thinks, if I really made an effort, think how much better I could do. Looking at the photo (right), ohhhh.... how can I let myself be so big?? Could I have surgery?? Liposuction??

Friday 15th Feb 2002

Bit of a crappy week for one reason or another. Valentines day was a dead loss, poor me!! Nobody loves me!

Slimming World Week 16

Slimming World Weigh-In
Today's weight =10 st 10 lbs (150 lbs)
Weight Lost = 2 lb
Weight lost so far = 16 lbs

Mon 18th Feb 2002

Another weighing in day, though I am very tempted not to go!! Today I am going to the Zoo with Judith and her 2. I am taking along my own food.

I cannot believe it, I lost 2 lb. I went to the Zoo (no this is not why I lost the 2 lb). And came home and because I had nibbled a bit I felt well, fat and was in 2 minds as to whether to go get weighed. I went and I AM SO GLAD I DID. I feel brilliant.

Sun 24th Feb 2002

We went to the cinema today to see Monsters Inc. I was very good and only ate a bit of popcorn. Ok, so we went for a meal afterwards. I had chicken salad and me and J shared a dessert, so I think all in all I was pretty good. Over the last week I have indulged in ermmm rather a lot of chocolate, stuff we got for the kids that sat in the fridge and just waited to be eaten. Ohhhhh chocolate is sooooo gorgeous cold. So, I do not deserve to lose weight this coming week. I had my joint injection last week so hopefully my knees and hands will improve and I might JUST MIGHT be able to get to the gym.

Slimming World Week 17

Slimming World Weigh-In
Weight = 10 st 8 lbs (148 lbs)
Weight Lost = 2 lb
Total weight loss = 18 lbs

Monday 25th Feb 2002

Yes, I get weighed again tonight. Why do they seem to come around so quickly, when I could do with that extra day or so to indo any damage I've done!!

Thursday 28th Feb 2002

As you can see I lost another 2 lb. I am SO pleased. I do feel though that I must be more careful with my eating, I am getting rather sloppy and not eating properly. It is bound to catch up with me!!!!

WEEK 18

(Still going to Slimming World!)

Monday 4th March 2002

I meant to go to the Slimming World meeting tonight but I felt I had put 2 lb on and was not in the mood to be told I had put weight on. I know I should have gone and what's a few lb compared to all I have lost so far. But honestly I could not face going. Also the kids were being a pain (R especially, she was crying not wanting mummy to go out). And N came home late. All this........well....

Wed 6th March 2002

I am going to be so good this week. I was good yesterday, well, till N came home then I opened a pack of cookies for the kids and ate 5 of them. Well at least they were small cookies. So that makes it a little better!!!! I have been trying on clothes and they are beginning to fit me better. It is so nice putting things on and finding they are not too tight!!!!

Saturday 9th March 2002

I found this GROSS photo of me taken around 1995/6. If I begin to feel fed up at this trying to lose weight, I will just take a look at this photo!!!!! The other person is my sister Vanessa (she has since put on weight, gone to slimming World and lost LOADS) and she is getting into size 14's. Because she was doing so well on Slimming World, this is why I decided to try it and I am glad I did. Judith has been following Atkins, I really don't know how she sticks to it, but she does. I was reading some old entries and she weighed 15 st 1 lb and when I spoke to her the other day she was at 14 st, so she has lost 14 lbs since November.! Tonight I am going to a 70's disco with Nicola. I will put up a piccy later!! Food is provided and you take your own drink (diet lemonade for me!), ok, so I admit it I might take along one teeny bottle of wine!?

This photo was taken about 1995/6 at my youngest sister's Hen Night

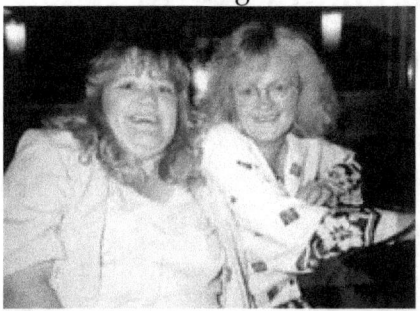

As you can see I look a bit thinner in the photo below!!!

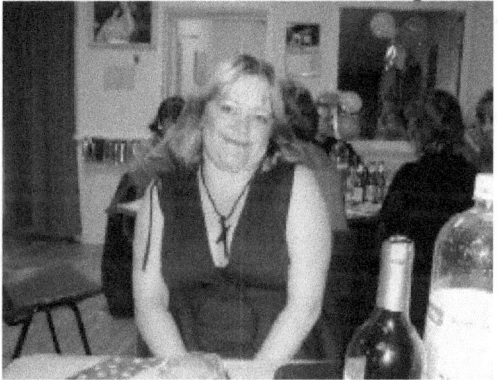

This photo was taken at the 70's disco March 9th 2002

NOTE

Ermmmm... I had a great time at the disco, such a good time, I ended up in casualty! I missed my teatime insulin, hadn't eaten since lunch and overdid the wine - all in all not a good combination for me. They kept me in till Monday morning, told me off and sent me home now that my bg's were stable. Here I am at the disco (note the wine bottle!), I was drinking diet lemonade too! I wished the dress hadn't been sleeveless (I hate sleeveless, hate my arms)

Slimming World Week 19

Monday 11th March to Sunday 17th March 2002

Ooops, as you can see I never wrote anything this week. Despite the fact that I went to Slimming World on Monday (11th March) and lost 3 lbs - YES 3 lbs.!!!!!!! I have not been on the computer much lately but will get going again on the web site seeing as I am losing this weight at last!!

Week 20 (Still at Slimming World!)

Slimming World Weigh-In
Today's Weight = 10 st 5 lbs (145 lbs)
Stayed the same
Total Loss So Far = 21 lbs

Monday 18th March 2002

Weigh-In tonight. I cannot stay to the class tonight cos I have a meeting at the school. Ah well.

Yesterday I went to Southport for the day and trudged round the shops all day (thus walking off a fair few calories!). I met N for lunch and I had a coronation chicken baguette but only ate half of it, is my stomach shrinking??? Actually stomachs do not shrink, they don't, you just get fuller on less food cos you are used to eating less. I got to my slimming club, rushed in (had to be quick as I had a meeting in my sons school). Hopped on the scales, and I had stayed the same. A little disappointing but I am glad I never put any on. I want to be under 10 st so badly (that's under 140 lbs). I went to the school and someone actually said "have you lost weight?". That is the first time anyone has said anything - well, N's work colleague Steve (Mmmm.....sexy Steve person) said a short time ago that I looked like I had lost weight (which spurred me on so much I can tell you!)

Wednesday 20th March 2002

I have good intentions I really do, it's just not always that easy to ermmm...follow them! R is off sch sicky, which easily drives me to the kitchen (often). And before you know it it's time to go for the next weigh-in!! And another 'wasted' week when I could've lost weight but didn't. Then the next week same etc etc. I DO NOT WANT THIS ! No crappy eating, no picking stuff I don't really want. Ok so it might be chocolaty and yummy and scrummy and there - but that is no excuse when you are trying to lose the weight you have had hanging around for far too many years.

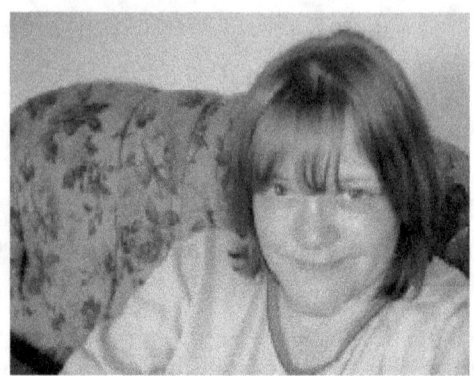

Here I am with brown hair, I like changing it!

Saturday 23rd March

I decided to try on a pair of frayed denim shorts that I bought ages ago (they would not go near me!). I bought them off the shop thinking they were size 18 (it said so on the hanger). But no, someone had put them on the wrong hanger and they were a size 14 (oh bugger...I thought at the time). Well, I got them off the bottom of the wardrobe and tried them on......wow, I got them on AND fastened (ok so I had to lie down on the bed)..but I ACTUALLY got them on!!! It is weird though, I still feel a size 18/20+, I can get into 16's comfortably and even the odd 14. I can see in the mirror that I am slimmer, but my brain has not quite caught up with the fact. I was wondering WHY...WHY did the denim shorts fit?? Why can I now get into that dress that was far too small/tight??? Actually it would help a great deal (help a MEGA deal) if more people actually noticed I had lost weight. I don't want loads of compliments but SOME comments would be nice?! Is it so un-noticeable??

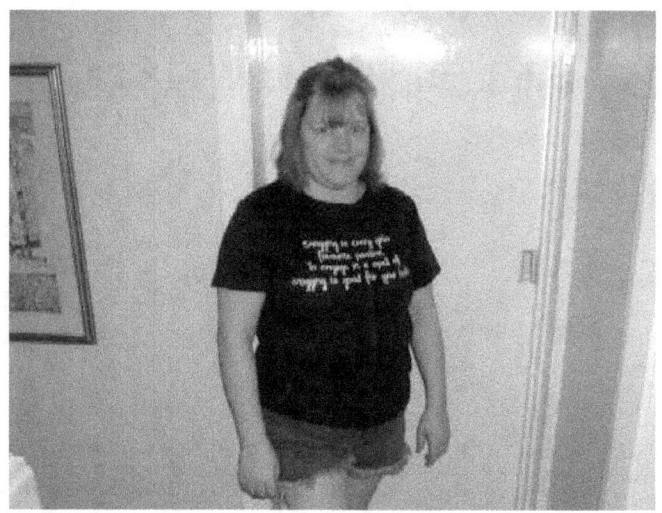

Not too self-conscious here!!

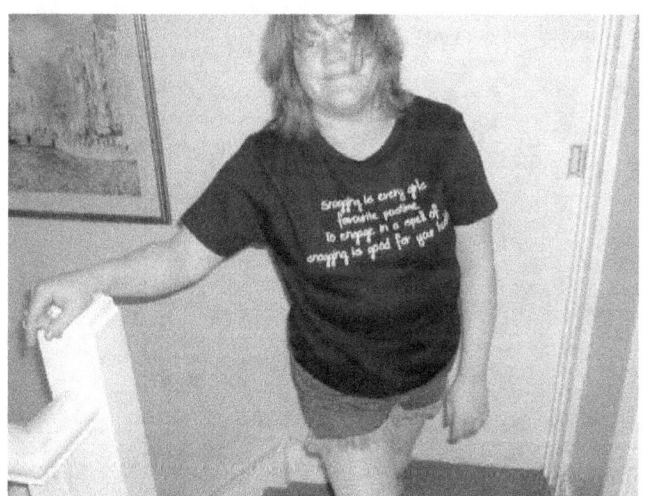

Still got a few spare tyres!!!

Slimming World Week 21

Slimming World Weigh-In
Today's Weight = 10 st 4 lbs (144 lbs)
Loss = 1 lb
Total loss so far = 22 lbs

Monday 25th March 2002

Yeah...I went to slimming world and I have lost another lb. I found 2 photos, old ones of me and took them in. They are truly GROSS photos. I think people were pretty amazed by the difference in me!!! I have put the photos in below for all to see. When you are slimmer you can put fat photos for all to see but when you are at the beginning and fat, you cannot put fat ones there! I can't anyway.

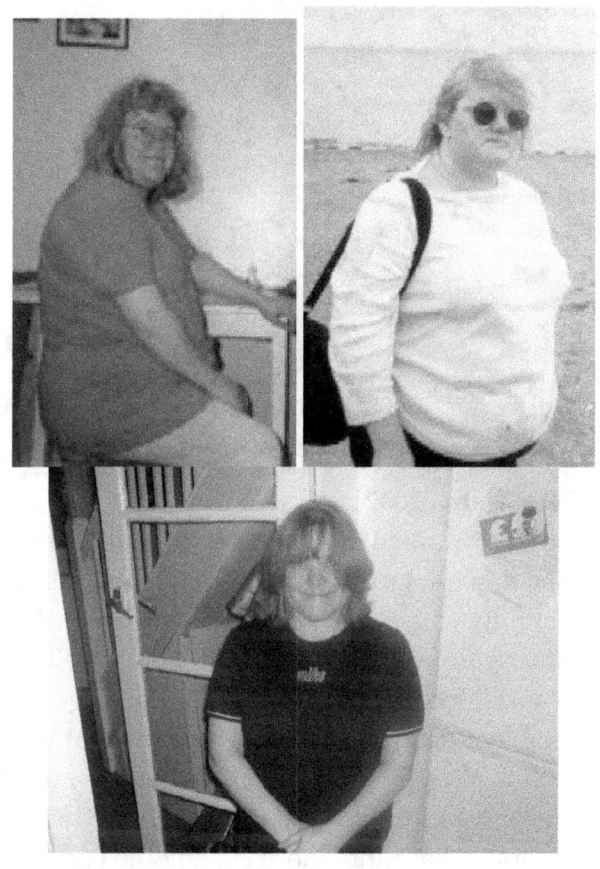

1st photo was taken in 1997 ermmm wow, I was so big (ok I was a bit pregnant, but still!). The 2nd photo was taken August 2001 (last Summer Holiday) AND I thought I was thinner then!!! I don't think so!!!! The 3rd was taken Monday March 25th 2002. It is so weird looking at these 3 photos!

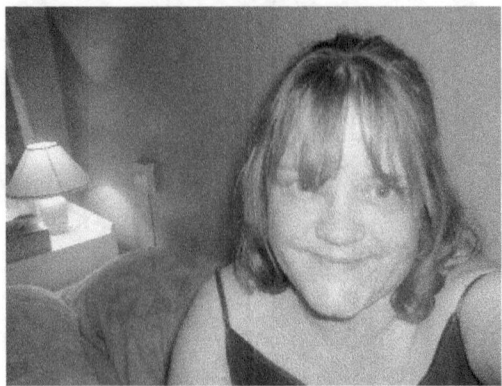

I am still very reluctant to have photos taken of the 'whole of me' because I feel I look lumpy/fat/big

Tuesday 26th March 2002

It's funny how some days are fat days and others aren't, or even thin days! I went out shopping today, in a pair of jeans (something which I never wear as a rule). I felt quite slim (slimmer anyway). trudged round the shops. Felt knackered, sure I looked knackered. The lighting in the shops is so harsh (I have said this before). Then....in a lot of the shops they have loads of teeny weenie clothes size 8's and 10's (I am a 16 with the odd 14 thrown in at the moment) There are loads of skinny people all around and well....by the end of the day I felt huge/fat. So what was a good day has turned into a fat day! But I have to remind myself of how I have done so far and LOOK at the photos above.

Thursday 28th March 2002

It is J's birthday today he is 11. Happy Birthday J. We took him and 2 friends to LaserQuest, they loved it. then we went to Pizza Hut, I was very good and had a salad (though there were probably hidden cals in the potato salad n coleslaw but still better than Pizza!) Oh I did have some (not all of R's ice-cream. Hi to Jennie who emailed me, she is also following the Slimming World plan (the first person I have met online who is doing Slimming World). She has done so well so far, having lost 22 and a half pounds since January.

Friday 29th March 2002

Everyone wants their Easter Eggs!!! I have been nibbling chocolate here and there but must not get too carried away! Actually I feel so yuck today, sore throat etc (kinda what R had - she has been so unwell, I was starting to get really worried and she has lost weight so I have been trying to tempt her with allsorts, even chocolate)

Saturday 30th March 2002

R had a bit of a bad night, hopefully she can get to see the doc today.

Sunday 31st March 2002

Went to my parents house today and my sister and her hubby were both amazed by my weightloss and mum and dad thought it was great too. At last!!! At last they have noticed. It has been ages (years) since I have worn jeans and if you are careful what you wear with them then you can look thinner than you are. N and I were going to go out and have a meal (I was SO looking forward to a HUGE steak - free on a red day!). But 1. The restaurant we like was totally booked till 9pm and 2. R was getting upset and just wanted to go home not to her nanas who was gonna baby-sit. J is staying in his other nanas in Flint. I was looking forward to going out, but ah well, maybe next time soon. So instead I ordered Chinese!!! You've gotta have a treat at Easter! I did over do the chocolate nibbling at my mums. I MOST DEFINITELY will not have a weightloss this week with one thing and another.

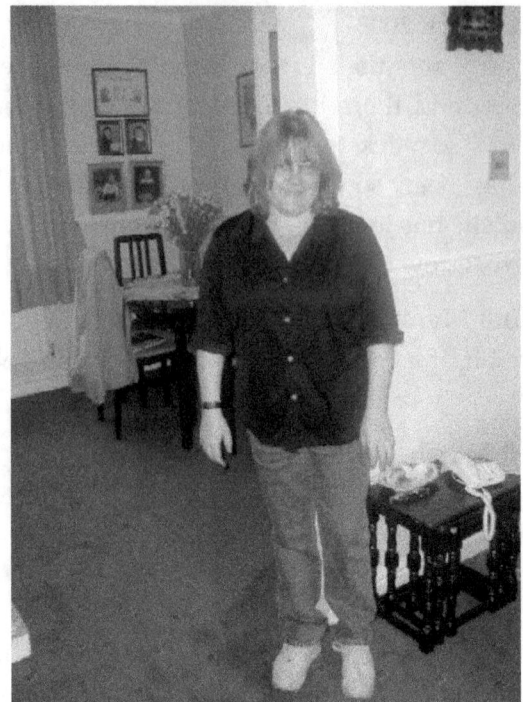

Taken today at my mum n dads

Slimming World Week 22

Slimming World Weigh-In
Today's Weight = 10 st 3 lbs (143 lbs)
Loss = 1
Total Loss So Far = 23 lbs

Monday 1st April 2002

It is my mums birthday today, Happy Birthday MUM. Yes. it is weigh-in day again. I do not know how I have done, but whatever, I am going to be SO good this week - like an angel!!!

Tuesday 2nd April 2002

Well, yesterday I went to get weighed and YES I lost another lb. I did not stay to the meeting cos I had booked a meal for N and I at Surfers for 6.30pm. It was N's birthday last Friday. I was quite good at the meal and suffered badly some hours later (I think I am allergic to spicy food?) I didn't have any alcohol! Today we (me and the kids) finished off the last of the Easter Eggs, now I feel thoroughly sick, really sick - serves me right! I know I have to be SO GOOD this coming week or I will most definitely put on weight next week.

Wednesday 3rd April 2002

I have printed out a set of charts for N to fill in, food diaries! I have done 10 weeks worth. It is time to get SERIOUS with his weight. He weighs (now he won't like me saying this) 19 st 8 lbs (274 lbs). He really really has to do something about his weight. Besides which I cannot stand the constant moaning about his weight (from him!).

Friday 5th April 2002

Well according to MY scales I have put on 1 lb and AND I feel fat - it's not fair!!! I do, I feel very fat today, bulgy fat, flabby fat, bloated fat. My 2 sisters came down and we talked dieting all the time, Nessa has been going to SW and now weighs 9 st 12 and a half pounds, I am 4 and a half lbs behind her! No it's not a race. We are all going to France in July, me, my 2 kids, Nessa, her 2 kids + hubby, Teresa and her 2 and her hubby and my mum and dad. We are all trying to lose them spare tyres now!!!. Teresa wants to lose about 10 lbs (yeah that's all) I think Nessa wants to lose 12+ and me, well I want to lose another 21 lbs.

I have been doing the weights each night and also I have been doing 100 ab-crunches each night. I am aiming to keep this up...well...till I get bored with it basically!!! I am hoping the ab-crunches help to even out or even flatten my stomach!

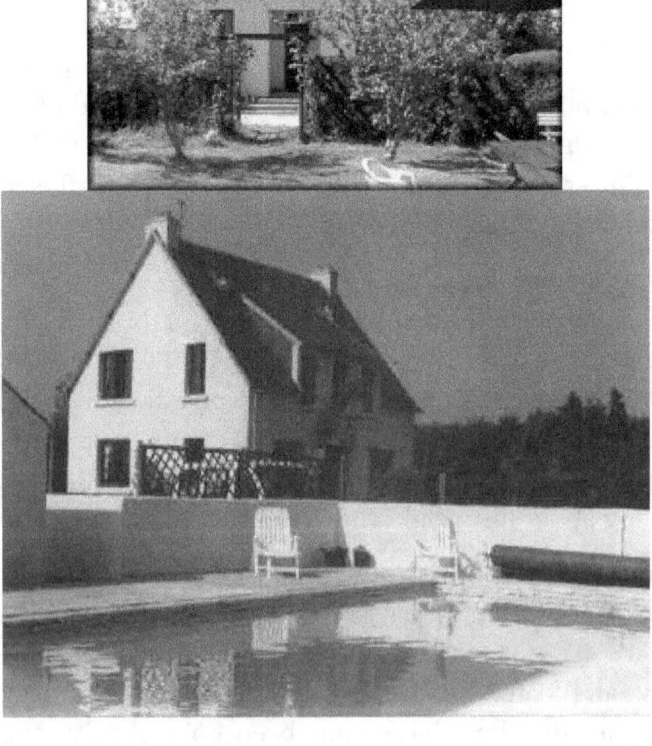

This is where we will all be staying on Holiday in July. It sleep up to 15 (there are 14 of us that includes the kids). It is called Coat Ailliss

Sunday 7th April 2002

Well, I have actually been counting my sins properly, I have been writing down EVERYTHING. Thanks to Jennie (my friend who is also following Slimming World, she has her own website-See Links Page), I have got back into counting, she is very careful about counting her sins and has done brilliantly so far with her weightloss only having had one gain of half a pound! We went to McDonalds yesterday, they have play tubes for the kids, J is too big for them really but he went in them to help his little sister. I was SO hungry (should have eaten before we went out) and had 2 plain burgers (no fries at least). So today I am having as few sins as possible. I had a very healthy start to the day - I had chopped banana/apple and a Muller lite yoghurt. We are off out later to Pekforton Castle and I am in the middle of cooking some chicken for some tasty sandwiches.

Slimming World Week 23

Slimming World Weigh-In
Weight This Week = 10 st 4 lbs (144 lbs)
Gain = 1 lb
Total Lost So Far = 22 lb

Monday 8th April 2002

I know, I just know I have put weight on this week! I have been feeling fat for the last week and it's my own fault. Now what did I eat??? Let me try and recall!!! Chinese takeaway/big meal out/chocolate eggs (lots and nibble of them too)/nibbles, nibbles, nibbles, pick, pick, pick. We shall see!!

As you can see I gained 1 lb. I know why I had a gain, because I have been picking n all that. I was not disappointed about gaining a pound, just annoyed with myself. I did the weighing last night, I weighed people as they came in which I enjoyed. Someone else was collecting the money. I did manage to tell one woman she had gained 10 lb (in 1 week) and I am sure I must have made her feel real sick. I had calculated wrong and she had lost not gained, so I felt quite awful!

Tuesday 9th April 2002

Today I have started counting my sins properly and I aim to stick to the correct amount for weightloss. I am going to eat sensibly all week. I do not want several weeks of getting nowhere and before you know it, it is holiday time! When you eat sensibly you don't feel hungry, or you shouldn't. Ok, so we all have times where we feel we need to eat loads (binge even) but as long as this is relatively rare!!

Wednesday 10th April 2002

Apart from half a mars bar I have been good today! The kids have gone back to school (now I miss them!). I am going to make a supreme effort to go to the gym on Friday, I want to get back into the routine of going twice a week.

Thursday 11th April 2002

Busy day in one way or another! Judith came round (she is now 13 st 11 lbs).

Saturday 13th April 2002

I have been very good counting sins and doing some exercise. I actually went to the gym yesterday!! I am so glad I went. I stayed almost 2 hours, but didn't overdo it! I have booked myself in for a fitness assessment next Friday and they will then do a programme for me. My very first fitness assessment was SO bad, I was in the bottom category, the 2nd one was slightly better. I am hoping to get back into the habit of going twice a week. I WILL be going in he morning, N will look after the kids I will go to the gym for 2 hours. They like to laze around on Sunday mornings so I will take the chance to go to the gym. Tomorrow if it is nice we plan to go for a walk on the hill, the kids will love that. N gets weighed in the morning, he has been doing well with the diet, a few blips here and there, but good for him.

Sunday 14th April 2002

Neil has lost 5 lbs this week and he lost 3 lb last week making 8 lbs altogether!!!! This is great. He is feeling good about dieting (with my help!)

Slimming World Week 24

Slimming World Weigh-In
Today's Weight = 10 st 1 lb (141 lbs
Loss = 3 lb
Total Loss So Far = 25 lbs

Monday 15th April 2002

Well, it's 5pm and I go get weighed in 2 hours. I feel I have done well the last week, I have eaten better. I went to my diabetic clinic and they are so pleased with my weightloss so far. I cannot weight (!) to break the 10 st barrier and be 9 st something. That will be fantastic, but I know I have not done it this week, hopefully next week. N has done so well and lost 8 lbs in 2 weeks. I am reluctant to put J (who is 11) on a diet but at my weightloss rate, I will weigh less than him soon. He needs to lose weight definitely, but hopefully if we get more active that will do the trick (and cutting out all the stodgy/sweets/cakes too many pizzas)

YES!!!! I lost 3 lbs. That's what you get for eating properly and counting 'sins'. I feel so much thinner!!

A BIG thank you to Leah O'Meara my Slimming World Consultant! She's been great, it's funny, I knew she had faith in me to lose weight from the first Slimming World meeting and I feel this has helped tremendously, from the very beginning I felt I COULD actually do it this time.

Slimming World Week 25

Slimming World Weigh-In
Today's Weight = 10 st 4 lbs (144 lbs)
Gain = 3 lbs
Total Lost So Far = 22 lbs

Monday 22nd April 2002

Can you believe it. I actually put on 3 lb. YES 3 lb. I knew I had put on weight cos my skirt felt so much tighter, so it wasn't a huge surprise, but I was not expecting to have put on 3 lb. I did go to Cadburys last week with Kim and ok I had a fair share (more than!) of chocolate over the week. On the other hand I did go to the gym 3 times so in a way I thought it would cancel out the chocolate (obviously not!)

Tuesday 23rd April 2002

I feel very determined to lose this weight so I am not going to let my gain bother me (well...ok, it does a little bit). I am going to count my sins this week and write them down, when I do this I am more successful. N has been doing so well, he has lost 11 lbs so far (in 3 weeks). I have been trying on different clothes. I am so used to wearing mostly black that it is difficult to wear brighter colours. Also, I have always worn long skirts and I feel self-conscious wearing shorter ones.

Thursday 25th April 2002

I have been eating well. I have bought a few clothes lately (off EBay), some nice strappy summer dresses. One is a size 16 and is slightly tight across my ermmm....chest and the other is a size 12 which is again only slightly tight across the same. Funny how sizes differ. Some 16's are too big, some too small.

Friday 26th April 2002

I keep making this cheese quiche (no pastry). I will end up looking like one!! It is sin free on the SW plan and really nice. Basically you get 2 tubs of cottage cheese, 1 tin of macaroni cheese, one chopped onion and 2 eggs, mix them all together and put in a flan dish or similar and bake for 30-45 mins. It's lovely hot or cold.

Saturday 27th April 2002

Went to my mum n dads for the day. Had a nice day though mum made too many sandwiches and I ate too many (even though it was ww bread) also she had a chocolate roulade and I had some.

Slimming World Week 26

Slimming World Weigh-In
Today's Weight = 10 st 5 lbs (145 lbs)
Gain = 1 lb
Total Lost So Far = 22 lbs

Monday 29th April 2002

I put another lb on. I go from being totally depressed about it to being SO determined to get back on track and get this weight shifting again. I am going to write down everything I eat this week, count all my sins - do it properly and have a weightloss next week.

Tuesday 30th April 2002

I have got to start eating properly, thinking about how I have been eating I realise I have been eating for convenience, i.e. eating food that take little or no preparation. Too much tinned stuff not enough healthy food

Wednesday 1st May 2002

Nessa my sister came down today, she is dieting too. She now weighs just over 10st (140 lbs). We are going to France in July and we both want to lose more weight before we go. I felt stressed later on in the day and ate 4 custard cream biscuits (must stop eating when stressed). I feel FAT again worse luck. N and I have decided to do some ab-crunches tonight and 5 mins on the bike and some weights. I know 5 mins is not much but it IS when you are not used to it!! We'll build it up. I have an ab-cradle, small weights and a bike so I ought to use them.

Friday 3rd May 2002

Went to my sisters house yesterday. I was so good. Though I did nibble on some chocolate raisins!!! What was I saying about using the home fitness stuff?? Well so far I have looked at it, looked at the weights and the bike and the ab-cradle. To be fair to myself I have a cold and feel yucky.

Saturday 4th May 2002

I have been so lazy today. I have eaten cheese n onion crisps all day (not a varied diet day to say the least). I ate so much chocolate last night, I wish I hadn't, in the end I felt sick and it messed up my bg's. Now I will have to be so good to minimise the damage for when I get weighed on Monday night.

I do not want to get back into the habit of eating crappily, I must be more disciplined. It is not SO hard to eat a healthy diet and why undo the weightloss I have so far PLUS it is only 10 weeks to my French holiday

Sunday 5th May 2002

I was SO hungry all day, every single minute of the day. My 4 yr old little girl kept saying "Mummy I want some chocolate" We didn't have any in (*Groan*). She kept saying it all day (she is too young for PMS and that time of the month chocolate craving?) We went to N's mums (nanas). Me, N, R and J. 'Sfunny really, when we got through the door and said out hellos we all ran for the biscuit tin!!!!! I, I must add, did not have even one biscuit, not a nibble. N did, he ate the ones R left on the table. Ok, I did have a choc ice and so did N and so did the kids. Poor Marie (N's mum) her house was attacked by us relatives on a food binge!!! I was SO good, I managed to get through the whole episode with just eating the choc ice (Ok so there was nothing else Marie had in that I wanted to eat). We didn't just go there to eat of course, it was a nice visit though I think Bill and Marie were relieved when we went!!!!

Slimming World Week 27

Slimming World Weigh-In
Today's Weight = 10 st 2 lbs or 142 lbs
Loss = 3 lbs
Total Lost So Far = 24 lbs

Monday 6th May 2002

YEAH! I lost 3 lbs. I feel better now! Today I went up to the village and helped with the Scouts May Day Fair. I was good but did have some candyfloss oh oh and when I got home I was SOOOO hungry and it is a Bank Holiday weekend and we haven't had a treat in ages and I just didn't feel like cooking and N persuaded me (! kind of) and and and ermmmmmm. Well, we had a Chinese takeaway. I was okish. I had some Beef in Blackbean sauce and a few small spring rolls and a few prawn crackers - that is all my sins rolled into one today (or lets call it a flexi-day)

Wednesday 8th May 2002

When you don't want to think about food it ends up being all you DO think about. Last night I actually did some ab-crunches, but only managed 70. I want to have a weightloss this coming Monday, I don't want to have put any on at all. I want to weigh 9 st something (i.e. under 140 lbs)

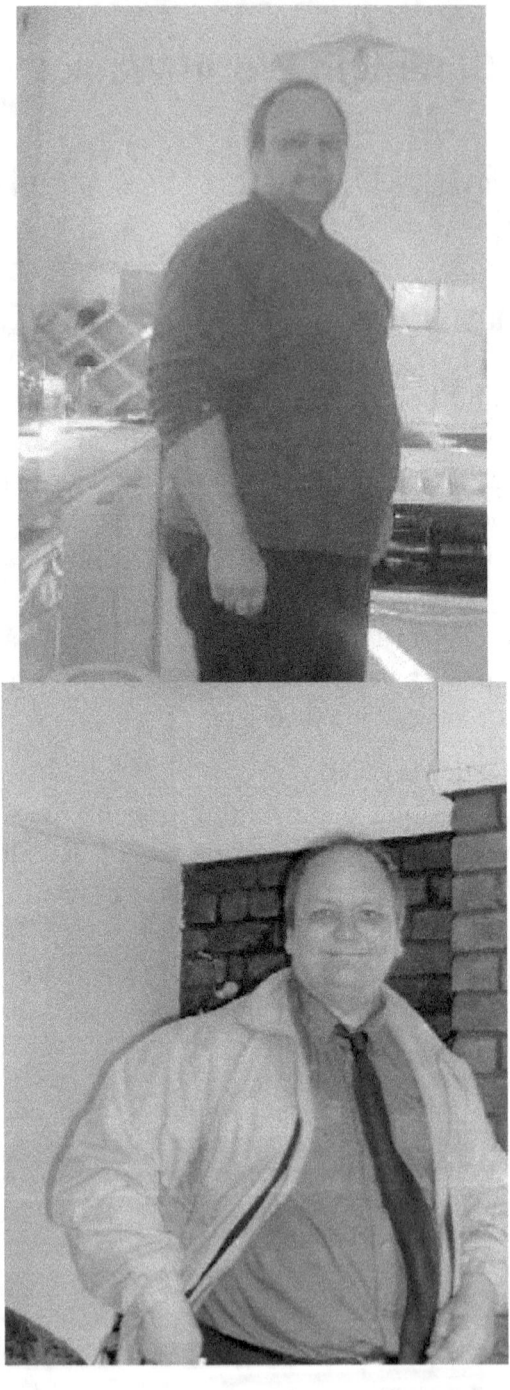

The 1st photo was taken in March 2002 and the 2nd in April 2002. N weighed about 19st 9 lbs (275 lbs)

N has decided that I can now start putting up some photos of him to show his weightloss. The first 2 photos were taken March/April and show what he weighed then, now he is already 13 lbs lighter. I will aim to take a new set of photos every time he loses 14 lbs - so keep a look out on his photos page. I think he is so brave, I know how much he EVEN hates having his photo taken in the first place. But I know with N, he will feel a lot happier when he gets to a weight he is happier at. I will do my best to help him as he helps me (he tells me off!!!).

N's Weigh-In Day
Weight = 18 st 7 lbs (259 lbs)
Loss = 3 lbs
Total lost so far = 16 lbs

Sunday 12th May 2002

Today we went to Norton Priory in Runcorn. We had a nice day out. To be healthier I made butties and in the priory I just had a coffee. But we did call at a pub on the way home and thought the main meal was slimming, I also had a dessert (strawberry sundae). N has done so well and has lost 16 lbs so far, I am so pleased for him, he is already looking slimmer and feeling it (I think!)

Slimming World Week 28

Slimming World Weigh-In
Weight = 10 st 3 lbs (143 lbs)
Gain = 1 lb
Total Lost So Far = 23 lbs

I knew I had gained weight. Never mind. I WILL do better and get back into losing more than gaining.

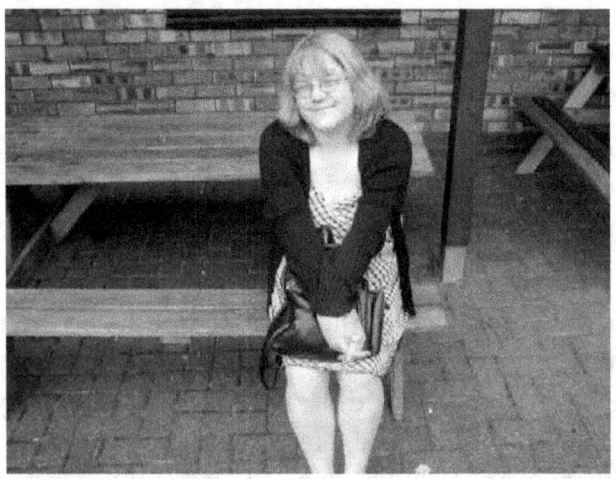

Monday 13th May 2002

This was me yesterday. We went out for the day to Norton Priory, it was a nice day (sunny) and we had a great time (lots of walking and seeing). We called at a pub on the way home (I had a ham/beef salad and a strawberry sundae - ok so I should've left the sundae!) For once I didn't spend the whole day thinking I was or looked FAT. It was too hot for a cardy at the beginning, but I must admit as soon as it went cold I grabbed the cardy and put it on (feeling the need to cover up!) Perhaps when I feel happier with the way I look, I will not need to cover-up? I am just about to go and get weighed. I feel as though I have put a pound or two on, in fact

I am sure I have?? Today I have eaten well (no picking so far!). I need to get more days where I do not pick. I need to make sure I write down in my book what I am eating and have a REALLY GOOD WEEK I knew I had put a lb on, but thank goodness it was only a pound and not more. I am going to have a good week and get this weight shifting (off)

Found a web site that allows you to see what you might look like with different hairstyles, now which one was the original?

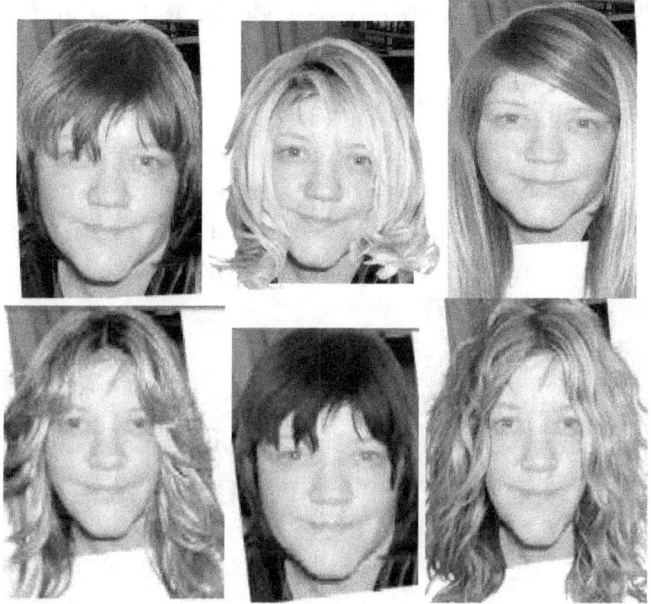

Tuesday 14th May 2002

Silly I know, but I found this other web site called ezface.com and you can send in your digital photo and after 24 hrs you get an email to say it is ready then you can go and 'try' on different make up. It is SO neat. You can go for the subtle look or the tarty look!!! You have a choice of foundations/eye shadows/eye liners/blushers and lipsticks, even nail polish, though this is on a models hand! It's a great way to try out new make-up looks.

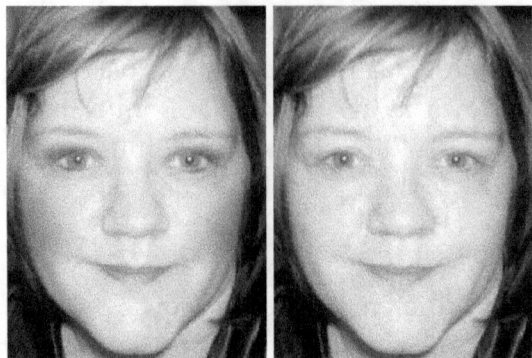

The first pic is with more make-up and the 2nd is with just foundation/eyeliner and lipstick!!!!!

Wednesday 15th May 2002

R is off with tonsillitis. I found myself nibbling children's dry chocolate cereal today, though this is all - so no too bad. Ooops and I ate R's chocolate bar, it was only a small one but gosh it was gone SO quickly and I hardly noticed I'd eaten it. And no - it wasn't worth it!

Why oh why do I pick so much???

Thursday 16th May 2002

I am going to eat healthily today, I really am. I have already done some weights (and it's barely lunchtime!! I weigh 143 lbs and I want to weigh under 140 as soon as poss (that's under 10 st) To be able to say I am 9st something will be great.

Sunday 19th May 2002

N has lost another 3 lb, making 19 lbs altogether, this is so great. he is doing so well and being really good and has loads of willpower! I wish I had the same! J is doing the Wirral walk today for Scouts, it is a 15 mile walk. He is raising money for his next Scout camp in July.

N's Weightloss

Today's Weight = 18 st 4 lbs (256 lbs)

Loss = 3 lbs

Total Loss So Far = 19 lbs

Slimming World Week 29

Slimming World Weigh-In
Today's Weight = 10 st 3 lbs (143 lbs)
Stayed the same
Total Lost So Far = 23 lbs

Monday 20th May 2002

I stayed the same weight, which is ok. I have got to crack this 10 st mark and get under it.

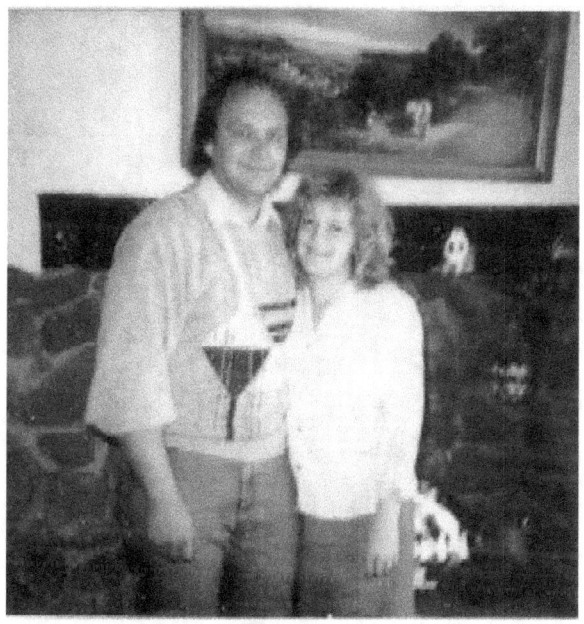

Cathy & N 1990 Pre-Children

Saturday 25th May 2002

Another picky week, when will I ever learn. I know that in order to lose weight I have HAVE to stop STOP picking. As you can see from my weightloss chart, I am getting nowhere. Ok, so I am pleased that I am not piling weight back on but, I am sure that's not too far away from being if I don't start eating healthier again. Scouts AGM today, with a bar-b-q n alcohol (not for me). I have already had my lunch so I know I will not be so hungry at the AGM, therefore not tempted to eat loads. I can have chicken or various other meats (not burgers, I hate burgers and I am not that keen on sausage at all)

I was very good at the bar-b-q, I just had one plain burger with onions. It was ok, wow there is 1 hunky Venture Scout Leader!!!!

Sunday 26th May 2002

N has lost another lb making 20 lbs so far, he is doing so well, he was convinced he had put on weight this week, neither of us has been particularly good.

N's Weigh-In

Weight This Week = 18 st 3 lbs (255 lbs)

Loss = 1 lb

Total Lost So Far = 20 lbs

Slimming World Week 30

(Oh my goodness 30 weeks have gone by!)

Monday 27th May 2002

Didn't go to Slimming World because I didn't feel well at all.

Tuesday 28th May 2002

Yes, this is the week I am going to be good and get losing the weight again. It helps when you don't feel too good of course, because then you don't particularly want to eat so much (yet!)

Sunday 2nd June 2002

The school had a Jubilee picnic on Friday. I went along to help. It was a hot day. At 3.30 J went with his class to Oaklands for the weekend, an outward bound course, me and R waved him off. I am trying to get a grip on the eating. I am vaguely following the red/green day plan for Slimming World, but I am not counting 'sins' properly. I bought a tin of shortcake biscuits for the kids and realised (when viewing the empty tin) that I had (give or take a few) more or less eaten the whole tin of biscuits. They are (were) small biscuits, too small in fact, but, I cannot believe I ate the whole lot (R only had a few)

Slimming World Week 31

Slimming World Weigh-In
Weight = 10 st 2 lbs (142 lbs)
Loss = 1 lb
Total Lost So Far = 24 lbs

Monday 3rd June 2002

We are getting weighed in the morning (this morning).

Well, I went to get weighed and I lost a lb. I am pleased, but I know that had I got weighed the usual time (tonight) then I would have most probably stayed the same weight (because you weigh 1 to 2 lb heavier in the night). Still, it's a loss and I have to see it that way and I WILL do better for next week. Neil is doing great, he has lost 22 lbs so far, he keeps losing every week. We both need to watch the picking though, it has been slipping back in.

Tuesday 4th June 2002

We went to see the Chuckle Brothers in Southport, it was fun. I did overdo the sweeties though! I did however have just fruit for breakfast (free). I have been having fruit and low fat yogs for brekky lately. We no longer buy white bread, always wholemeal now (even the kids will eat just this). all in all I am eating far less bread, which I'm sure helps.

Friday 7th June 2002

Someone has stomped on my hands, they are hurting so much (I have PA, psoriatic arthritis) and at the moment it's a total pain. Well, aside from this. I have been good for the last 2 days, feeling like crap does take the edge off your appetite! I have stuck to my sins yesterday and today and that makes me feel I am back on track (at long last). Maybe now I can crack this 10 st barrier. I realise I might get to Mondays weigh-in and not do so well, since apart from being good last 2 days, before that I was not so good. BUT....but....I will stick to it, think more about what I am eating, keep track of what I am eating so that the following week IT SHOWS!!

Saturday 8th June 2002

We ended going out for the day to Manchester Aviation Park (get the kids out!). It was rather good, made me want to hop on a plane and go somewhere (anywhere) though. Ate crap all day, as you do when you are out, unprepared.

Sunday 9th June 2002

My hands are so painful. It would (in an ideal world) make dieting easier. You know, difficult to eat n all that. But no. N got weighed, he has lost another lb. This is great. We ate crappily last week so we are gonna have a good week and both be in the next stone down.

Nothing fits me. I have had a 'trying on' session. Got loads of stuff out of my wardrobe and non of it fits. WHY? I feel as though I have put on a vast amount of weight. I now feel FAT at this weight, I know it is time to move on. I have been catching sight of myself in shop windows (reluctantly) and all I see is a short FAT person. I can bear looking at individual parts of me, say, an arm here, a leg there, even (arrgghhhhhhh) the odd glimpse of my stomach (only if held in). BUT but when I catch a look at the whole of me, I cringe. How HOW come I look so huge all of a sudden when I was looking slimmer?????? This is not just a FAT day, this has been creeping in for weeks. I know the answer, I need to get losing weight again, regularly, even small amounts. I need to be 9 st something not 10 stone something. I don't have far to go to be 9 st something. Then of course I want to be 8 st something (and AND maybe even 7 st something). Why in heavens name did I ever moan when I weighed 7 st 12 (110 lbs)??????? (ok I was in my teens then). So here I am 142 lbs (10 st 2 lbs) and I want to be a minimum of 120 lbs (8 st 8 lbs) so I still have 22 lbs to lose.

Slimming World Week 32

Slimming World Weigh-In
Today's Weight = 10st 5 lbs
(145 lbs)
Gain = 3 lbs
Total Lost So Far = 21 lbs

Monday 10th June 2002

Ooohhhh another weigh-in day (night). I wonder how I will have done? I hope at the least I have just stayed the same. PLEASE, PLEASE, PLEASE.

Well I got to my meeting. I have changed to morning ones, mainly cos it is easier with N. And I am not going to get depressed, not at all. I gained 3 lb. I knew I had. And N very kindly said to me (before the meeting)...." You'll hate me for saying this..." So I said " Go on, what?" and he said "You look fatter"

So, here I am (it's now 20 past 10 in the evening). I had my meeting at 9.30 this morning. I slept all day (had strong painkillers off the doctors for my joints). Ah, this is why I have eaten very little all day! Seriously, I have been good today, I have eaten sensibly, I even managed (with N's help) to make a corned beef quiche (sin free) this morning for my lunch. I have not overeaten nor eaten things I didn't mean to. And AND I am going to keep this up ALL week. I am going to stick to the Slimming World Plan and lose this weight (especially what I just gained!!!) But....OK....I still feel fat but not defeated!!

Tuesday 11th June 2002

Another day feeling crap. I did it, I got through yesterday with no nibbles, no cheating, no extra stuff. I am going to do the same today (so far so good here at 4 in the afternoon)!! N made me noodles for lunch.

Wed 12th June 2002

Another good day yesterday. I stuck to the plan. I am hoping to manage a whole week of it!!!!!! N is sticking to it too.

N and I need to relax more

Friday 14th June 2002

Another good few days. I am pleased with how I am doing. I wish I didn't feel SO fat though. Kathy if you are reading this - are my mails getting through to you?? Kathy is my friend and diet buddy in Ohio, we speak on the phone. She is following the Body For Life Programme. Well, I hopped on the scales (here at home) this morning and have not lost a thing, this made me feel awful. I got a few summer things off EBay for my hols, oh they fit ok, but I feel I look gross in them. I WANT TO BE SLIM - SLIMMER. !

Sunday 16th June 2002

Went to the Commonwealth Games Athletics Trials in Manchester.

Slimming World Week 33

Slimming World Weigh-In
Weight This Week = 10 st 3 lbs (143 lbs)
Loss This Week = 2 lbs
Total Loss So Far = 23 lbs

Monday 17th June 2002

Well here I am again, another weigh-in day and another week closer to the France holiday. I am SO looking forward to going to France and I am not going to let my extra lbs bother me (much!!!!!). I am glad I am lbs slimmer than I was last year at least.

Tuesday 18th June 2002

YES!!!!! I lost 2 lb. I am SO glad. On the way into the meeting I met the evening consultant Leah (whose classes I used to go to). She gave me a little pressy (for the times I did the weighing-in for her). She said she was leaving Slimming World, her and her family were going to live in Spain. Everyone will miss her. I owe my 1 st 9 lbs weight loss to her. I know I will do well with Carole (the morning consultant) she is very nice too. Yesterday at the meeting we all had to take in picnic stuff. I made a Lemon Cous Cous cake which was very nice, I got it off another girl's web site who is also following Slimming World. (Her web site is called Slim For Free and it's http://www.slimforfree.co.uk . Anyway, there was some good ideas for food to take on a picnic. Nessa came down (sister). She said she weighs 10 st (140 lbs) and wants to be 9 and 1/2 stone (133 lbs) for the French holiday. I guess 7 lbs in 3 weeks is ok if you really really try.

Friday 21st June 2002

Yikes! I have not updated for a few days! How have I been?? Well I started the week off well and stuck to my 'sins'. I have been writing down all I eat (it's on the fridge door). But today I was a total pig. I ate so much chocolate, it makes me feel sick thinking about it. In fact, that's all I have eaten tonight (no food) now this could be minimising the damage or just stupid?? I am going to York on a day trip tomorrow (on a coach with J). I am going to prepare my food for the day tonight. I am aiming to have as little as possible sin wise tomorrow, and so lots of walking. trouble is it doesn't help that my joints are knackered at the moment (very hurting). I am waiting for a phone call from the hospital so I can go and have a depo medrone (steroid) injection in my bum to sort my joints out, especially with the holiday coming up. I really don't know how I will do with my weigh-in on Monday, all I can do is as little 'damage' as possible between now and then. Don't you just wish you could turn back the clock and not do those dumb things!!

Slimming World Week 34

Slimming World Weigh-In
Today's Weight =10st 3 lbs
(144 lbs)
Gain = 1 lb
Total Lost So Far = 22 lbs

Monday 24th June 2002

Another weigh-in day. I hope I have lost some more weight. Only 3 more weigh-ins till we go to France.

Wednesday 26th June 2002

AS you can see I gained a lb this week. I feel a bit fed up about it but am determined to get the weight shifting again (that's the spirit!). So, I have been writing down everything I have been eating and really sticking to the plan. I did better than N, he gained 3 lb this week. He has a splurge on wine last week and overeating. He is trying to be good now. It's been an awkward time, I have not been so well (my joints have been very bad this time) and N has been off work helping me cos I have felt so ill. The hospital have faxed a steroid jab through to my docs, but typical them, they cannot do it till NEXT Thursday. I have found a place online that is a great help with slimming support, there is a link on my front page. It's called Slimming World With Fun2 (it's on MSN groups). There's lots of people on it, it has loads to offer.

Sunday 30th June

N has lost 2 lb this week, which is good. He rather overdid the wine and nibbles lately (stress!).

N's Weightloss

Weight this week = 18 st 1 lb (253 lbs)

Loss = 2 lbs

Total lost so far = 22 lbs

Slimming World Week 35

Slimming World
Weigh-In
Today's Weight = 10 st 2 lbs
Loss = 2 lbs (yippee!!!)
Total lost so far = 24 lbs

Monday 1st July 2002

This weigh-in and the next weigh-in before the France holiday!

Wow I am so glad I lost weight this week. A whole 2 lbs, perhaps this is the start of a new downward slide! Ok, so I have a holiday coming up and the potential to put some back on, but still. I would truly love to be under 10 st for the hols but that means I have to lose 3 lb by next week (possible).

Sunday I went along to my sister's christening (well her baby's). It was ok, a bit of a chore in that my hands and feet were killing me unfortunately. I ate very little (good old me!). Had to listen to my 2 sisters (+ their hubbies) and the friend and her hubby (who are coming along too) all talking about how much alcohol they can get in one visit to the hypermarket on the first day in France. And in the other ear, my mum was busy telling everyone how CATHY (me) cannot drink AT ALL, not a drop. Ok, so alcohol does not agree with me at present (must be the drugs I am on)!. But to stamp on my chance of even a few glasses - honestly, what are parents like? I am looking forward to going to France (wish I could lose 14 lbs between now and the 13th July when we go, but still at least I am 1 st 10 lbs (24 lbs) lighter than I was on holiday last year.

Tuesday 2nd July 2002

Have been good today (it is now 4.15pm). I have already packed a few things away for the holiday. I have a few items of clothing that I wonder whether to pack or not, seeing as they are too tight, probably better to leave them at home really.

11 days to go to the France holiday!

Thursday 4th July

Had my steroid jab today (at last), so I hope my joints will settle down now. Wandered round the village after my jab and met a neighbour for a coffee. She insisted on me having a scone, so I had half but scraped off half a pound of butter first!. had my lunch date with Andy (my twice a week lunch liaison!), actually it's one of the parents from preschool, who kindly offered for me and R to go there for lunch on Tues and Thurs cos R is on a split day at preschool and it saves me walking all the way home and back in an hour (he lives near the school).

Sunday 7th July 2002

There's nothing like a good old 'trying clothes on' session right before your holiday to make you feel FAT. Yes. I've gone through my holiday clothes and YES they all make me feel FAT, not just a little bit, A LOT. I have 'spare tyres' where I thought they had gone. I have lumps and bumps that I thought had at least flattened a tiny bit (but haven't). I have t-shirts that I thought fitted me but don't. I have dresses that were going to fit me (but don't). I have smoothish skin (courtesy of hair removal!) but too much skin!!!! AND AND I have 5 days YES 5 days in which to change all this (I wish). Ah well. I suppose I had better think positive, I am 24 lbs lighter than last years hol, I am going to France and I have another holiday to look forward to in August (with N and the kids in Norfolk Broads). Wish I hadn't tried those clothes on though.

Slimming World Week 36

Weigh-In
Weight This Week = 10 st exactly (140 lbs)
Loss = 2 lbs
Total Lost So Far = 26 lbs

Monday 8th July 2002

I am so pleased to have lost 2 lb this week. I think I deserve it, I have been counting those 'sins'. I have not got under 10 st but to be this low (haven't been this in years) is GREAT. I really enjoyed today's meeting, I enjoyed weighing people and I won Slimmer of The Week and got a huge bag of lovely fruit. I bought the latest Slimming World magazine and will read this bit by bit.

Wednesday 10th July 2002

Am having a very bready day, ok so it's ww bread so perhaps not quite so bad, but I have already over done it. Still, I am making a corned beef quiche (FREE) for tea and did ok with lunch etc. I am looking forward to going to France on Friday but could do with it being another week away - not for more weightloss but to try and get 'un-tired'. (Somehow)! I know the hol will be hectic.

Slimming World Week 37

13th July to 21st July(on holiday)

Well I am on HOLIDAY in France this week, hopefully enjoying the sunshine.

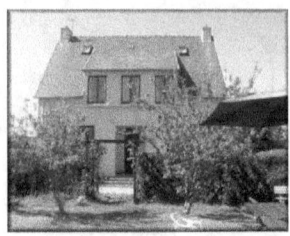

This is where we are staying (me, my 2 kids, my 2 sisters and their hubbies and their children and a neighbour of my sisters with his wife and little girl - that's 14 of us altogether), in one big house, it has it's own pool, orchard, games room, sauna/jacuzzi etc and looks lovely on the web site. I hope it is in 'real' life!!

I am hoping to wear my summery clothes (having lost lbs so far).. I have taken a one piece swimming costume (would've loved a red one, but have stuck with good old 'slimming' black!. I also bought a 2 piece but dunno if I will wear it (perhaps if no one is around/it's dark/or I am in a don't care mood), N says I do not look fat in it, but well....... I have a few pairs of shorts and lots of t-shirts. I know there is a beach about 20 mins walk away from where we are staying (ohh and a nudist beach nearby too - !) I shall miss N (since he is not going, but staying at home, going to work). I have never been on a ferry before. We sail from Plymouth and get to the other side (Roscoff?) 6 hours later..

I will be back doing my website as soon as I get back from my hol and I will be straight back to Slimming World. See the PHOTOS later (I hope!)

Slimming World Week 38

(After the Holiday!)

Slimming World Weigh-In
Weight = 9 st 13 lbs (139 lbs)
Loss = 1 lb
Total Lost So Far = 27 lbs

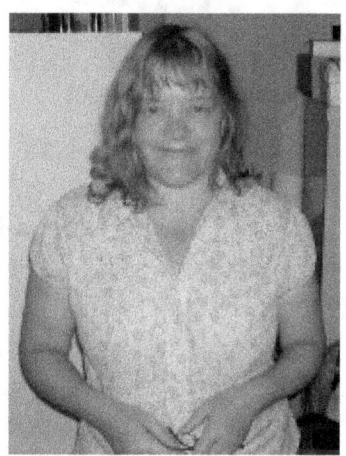

Here I am last night

Monday 22nd July 2002

Well here I am after my week in Brittany France and it's my weigh-in day! The photo below (and right)was taken yesterday (Sunday), I was trying to show off my tan and to show that I perhaps haven't gained too many pounds from the holiday!! I HOPE! It is almost time to go get weighed.

YES! I have lost a pound. I have had a weeks holiday in France and lost a lb!!!!!!!!!! I am now in the 9 stones, where I have wanted to be for a long time. I want to get under 9 st, so basically I need to lose another 14 lb or more. I will have to be good this week so any chocolate eating I did on holiday does not catch up with me.!!!

Tuesday 23rd July 2002

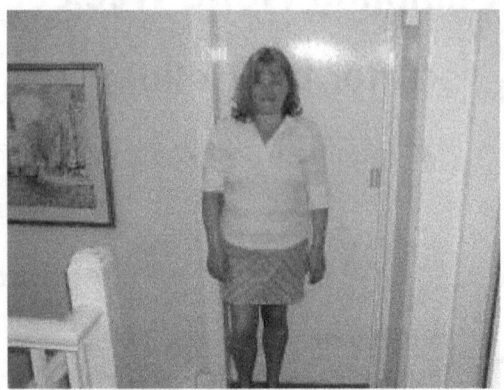

Still got a few 'spare tyres' to get rid of boo hoo!

Wednesday 24th July 2002

Went to the cinema to see Scooby Doo. Went with Judith and her 2 and my 2. I was SOOOOO good in the cinema,, no nibbles at all. Then went and had a Hawaiian (?) pizza afterwards and ate my fair share of smarties. And last night N and I went to the cinema to see Jason X (kinda boring) and I managed to have a hotdog, a bite of a mars bar and some MORE chocolate. Yes Cathy this will help you get your 2 stone award on Monday NOT. Who can I blame?? Ermmmmmmm.....just me unfortunately. Why do you have to have nibbles when you go to the cinema?? Well, I did ok during Scooby, just had a coffee, Judith's fault she took me into Pizza Hut afterwards.

Friday 26th July 2002

School hols are NOT good times to be trying to diet really. Take today. I went to the cinema again (thanks Judith) we saw Ice Age. I had a few nibbles, we ate out a Wimpy (I had a bacon and egg bap). I know it's all stuff I can count in but it's slightly off plan and I know I have gained a lb so far this week, I just know I have.

Saturday 27th July 2002

I am trying to be good, I am, really truly. I had this photo taken the other might in a dress that I kind of like but which is FAR too tight for me. I may not look huge in this dress but believe me I look SOOOOOO lumpy in it. If the camera catches you at a good angle it doesn't half make a difference. On the other hand I have lost count of all the GROSS photos of me where the camera has made me look absolutely enormous. I want to be able to get into this dress and be relatively lump free - then throw the dress away HA!

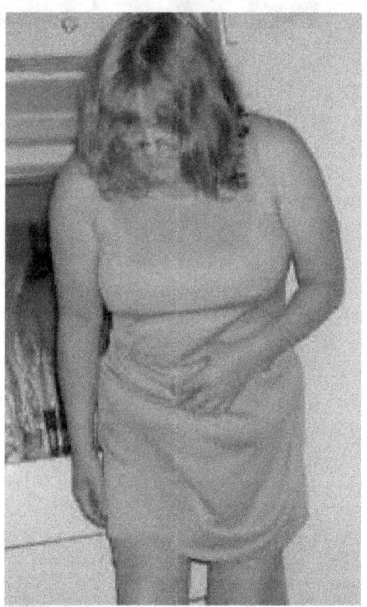

Sunday 28th July 2002

Had a great day out, a trip on a canal boat. We were on the boat for 2 hours then got off at a pub then had Sunday lunch (plus a few beers) then got back on the boat and came back again. It was boiling hot all day. Here I am with my friend Nicola on the canal boat (I am the one on the right)

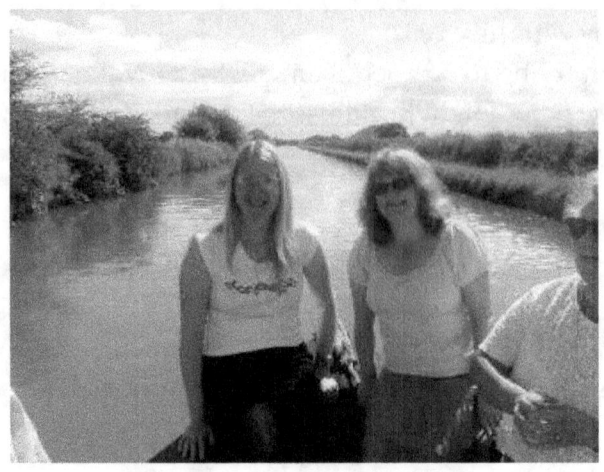

3 Weeks To Next Holiday. 12 Weeks To Christmas

Slimming World Week 39

Slimming World Weigh-in
Weight = 9 st 13 lbs
stayed the same
Total Loss = 27 lbs

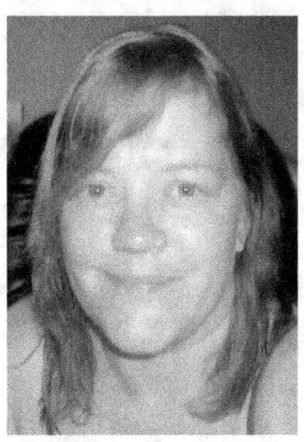

Monday 29th July 2002

Wonder what I will weigh today, since I ate so crappily last week. I so wanted my 2 st award this week. We shall see. It is 8.20am and at 9am I go get weighed. I know I have put on weight, I have eaten so much with going out this last week. So I get a few steps further away from my 2 st award yet again. I really want to make an effort this coming week, I want that award!!

I am feeling rather fed up at the moment, well very fed up actually.....totally mega fed up. In the kind of the mood where I don't know what I want to do and can't be bothered anyway. I cannot believe I stayed the same, I am so pleased. Not long for our Norfolk holiday, can I be 9 st 7 lbs for it (133 lbs)? Would be nice, that's 6 lb to lose in 3 weeks.

Tuesday 30th July 2002

I have been digging out old photos from the attic, they are so painful to look at!! I look so HUGE in them really I do. The 1st photo was about 1997. The 2nd was last year on hol in Brixham. The 3rd photo was taken the other day on the canal boat trip (28th July 2002)

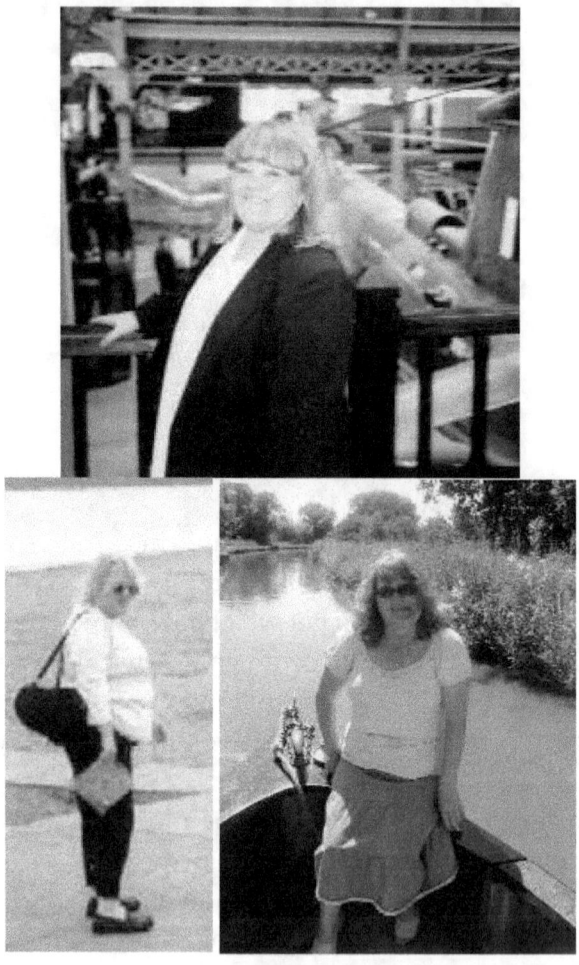

Have been very good today (so far). It is so tempting though (especially when you are fed up etc) to go into the kitchen and get something to eat, anything to eat.

Wednesday 31st July 2002

'When she was good she was very very good but when she was bad she was......' remember this rhyme? Well that's me at the moment. I am being very very good, too good. What will break it I wonder! I am feeling positive (good good), I am not overly hungry (even better) but.....God why do I have to look for a downside? There's gotta be one right? I am fed up of this eating lark. If I wasn't diabetic, well, it would be different - I would not have to eat. Not that I could like stop eating, no. I just perhaps wouldn't bother so much sometimes. It's hard to keep an even attitude towards food and how you feel about it all when you are desperately trying to lose excess weight. Food should be something you eat, enjoy and not think TOO much about. No problem. No, food is a bit of a problem (hence the weight problem). I know, I know I am losing weight (look ten times better) but don't you just get FED UP of the whole thing! I can't 'give up the ghost', not this close to getting to my ideal weight (have around 18-20 lbs to go), I would never forgive myself. But it's like the closer I get to where I want to be, the more bored I am with it all.

Sunday 4th August 2002

I went to the gym today, have not been for ages. I really enjoyed it, I stayed about an hour. I should make an effort and go at least once a week while the kids are off school, a weekend day is good since N is off. Then when R goes back to school I will go 2 or 3 times a week (if my joints will hold out!). The main problems I have at the moment are with my hands.

Slimming World Week 40

Slimming World
Weigh-In
Weight = 9 st 11 lbs (137 lbs)
Loss = 2 lbs
Total Loss = 29 lbs

Monday 5th August 2002

I really don't know how I will do on the weigh-in today. I feel I have eaten badly this week (as in over done it). The more I try to get this last 1 lb off to get my 2 st award the more I sabotage my efforts.

N - I am truly sorry, I cannot change things, I cannot turn back the clock - I wish things were different.

I AM sorry.

I want to lose this weight so much and I am glad I went to the gym yesterday, I can see myself getting hooked again, it is such a great stress reliever. I bought an Adidas t-shirt, very lycra, very size 18 (ooohhh too big I'm sure) NOT. All I can say is, don't they make lycra things SOOOO small. No way could I exercise in that t-shirt, it is double layered (more holding in effect!?) and would make you sweat like nothing else (perhaps this is the desired effect?) I reckon it would be comfy on a size 12 person. I am in a 14-16 at the moment. It gets you down though, buying something so BIG (18's are too big for me now) and whoa they are too tight. Bloody lycra - lycrap I think! Guess it's back to the sexy baggy t-shirts!

WOW MEGA WOW - I lost 2 lbs, I got my 2 st award at last!!!! YES YES YES this is fantastic. I hopped on the scales and was so convinced I had gained a little weight. It is a fantastic feeling to be losing the weight and to be doing it without it being too hard. I am eating well, not starving or denying myself stuff I like and yet I am losing weight. A big difference is that I no longer pick. OK, so I do sometimes (I am just human). But I am finding Slimming World so great, so easy to follow and it is getting to be my way of eating now - I am eating healthier than ever before.

Wednesday 7th August 2002

The kids stayed at my mum and dads last night. N and I did not know what to do with ourselves, so we finally did what we really wanted, EAT. Eat in peace, without interruptions, on our own. N had a meeting so I went along with him, so the evening started off innocently enough. After that we thought Mmmm why don't we go for a stroll along the prom (prom of sorts in WK). It was 10pm. Oh I was hungry. The people we visited said "Oh no children for the night.. you should go for a drink". Nah, we weren't in the mood for a pub so... what could we do first... we went to the chippy (Mmmmm fish and chips for Neil , chips and peas for me). We sat in the car on the prom to eat them. We did not eat ALL of them (so felt saintly!) Then we went for a walk, I am sure I walked off at least a few chips??? So did we get back in the car and go home??? NO. We strolled passed the shops, window shopping at 11pm is peaceful, ahhhhhh.... a shop was open, so... so... just a few packets of sweets. Indulged in these at home... went to bed (full) and guilty. And if I am entirely honest I did contemplate hanging over the loo (toilet) forcefully heaving up all the things I had not planned to eat. I did not do it. These times lately when I have overeaten it is very tempting to well... go puke. I am ashamed to say I have done this in the past. I hope that by being sensible and allowing myself 'treats' and so what if I overdo it sometimes, that I will not resort to doing dumb things. It's a bit like a panic thing really though, the more I see how well I am doing the more stressed I feel about the prospect of putting any weight back on.

Thursday 8th August 2002

I have been good today despite the fact that the kids made cakes and ok, I had to try them, but only small bit. I hopped on the scales in the bathroom... holy thingies... it said 9 and a half stone (oh my god have I lost THAT much?) I almost stopped breathing. It was slightly possible yes. BUT... but. I peered down at the dial (when I was off the scales) and some mysterious person (e.g. my son or daughter) had moved the dial so it was not set at the correct starting position. Oh it was brief, very brief but... made me go away and think twice about 'picking'.

Friday 9th August 2002

Judith came round today and we as usual talked about food, well, a bit. I had made a corned beef quiche (and we ate a little). It is so much easier to eat well when you have the stuff in. I have in some yummy grapes and Muller yoghurts (have about 10 yogs in the fridge). 18 lbs that is what I want to lose to be the weight I want to be. Doesn't sound like a lot at all does it?? That will take me to 8 and a half stones (have said this before) that's 119 lbs. I still don't like the way I look at the moment. I took loads of piccies the other night and deleted all of them (I looked so well... fat).I know, compared to how I was I look great but still not how I want to look. When I stop cringing when I catch sight of myself, this is when I will be fine.

Saturday 10th August 2002

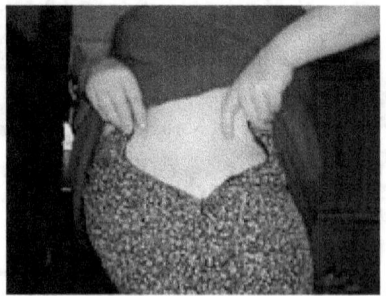

11th Feb 2002 (152 lbs)

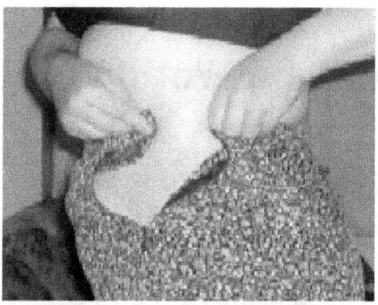

10th August (136 lbs)

Personally I do not see much of a difference, ok, so the skirt IS getting nearer to fastening but it is still miles away from fitting me.

Sunday 11th August 2002

It is my birthday next Sunday (*groan*), I will be ermmm ok 39. We go away on holiday on the 17th (day before my birthday) - that will give people an excuse for forgetting it (boo hoo), who says birthdays don't matter when you get older, of course they do.

N got weighed yesterday morning and has gained a lb. Now I am sure to follow suit tomorrow!! We went out for lunch today and had pizza (which I rarely eat as I am not a big fan of it). I declined the ice-cream and chocolate sauce!! Aren't I good!!

Slimming World Week 41

Slimming World
Weigh-In
Weight this week = 9 st 12 lbs (138 lbs)
Gain = 1 lb
Total Lost So Far = 28 lbs

Monday 12th August 2002

Ok, weighing day again and I am sure VERY SURE I have gained a pound, even 2. No panic if I have, I shall have a good week before I go on holiday and aim to be relatively active while on holiday!! (To a point)

Ok, so I gained a lb. I am not too bothered (much!) So I am going to stick to the plan this week, have a good holiday and get weighed in Slimming World on the Bank Holiday Monday (26th August)I know that I can do it. Well, other than getting weighed today has been rather boring (have managed to stop the kids from killing each other so far!).

Saturday 17th August 2002

Going on holiday today, I am looking forward to a week in the Norfolk Broads. I hope that we have at least half decent weather!!!!!!

Slimming World Week 42

Monday 19th August to Sunday 25th August

Well, I went on holiday on the 17th August for 1 week to the Norfolk Broads, hopefully I am having a GOOD time and the weather (yes the British weather) is being kind. It is my BIRTHDAY on the 18th August. Fancy having a birthday and a holiday away all rolled into one! If any two things are designed to help you put weight on, well, I don't know what is!!

See you all when I get back!

My next weigh-in (urgghhh after the holiday) is Monday 26th August - see Week 43. And then we have Christmas to aim for!)

Sunday 25th August 2002

Back From The Holiday!!

Well here I am back from my holiday. I had a great time and ate FAR TOO MUCH!!

Slimming World Week 43

Slimming World Weigh-In
Weight = 9 st 11 lbs
Loss = 1 lb
Total Loss = 29 lbs

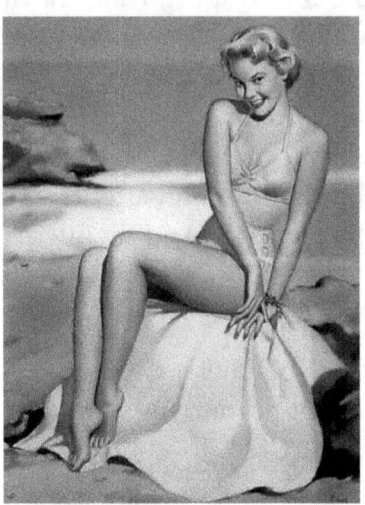

How I would have liked to look on my holidays
(in my dreams!!)

Monday 26th August 2002

Am I ready to be weighed again after my holiday? NO. I really had a great holiday and I got to meet my online friend Jennie who is also following Slimming World. She (and her family) came to visit us at our chalet camp and we had a lovely day out then she invited us to her home at the end of the week. We took lots of photos and I am hoping to get in touch with Slimming World magazine when we both get to our targets - who knows, you may see us featured in the magazine!!

Oh my goodness I lost a lb!!! HOW? HOW? I ate SOOOOOO much ice-cream and other stuff I don't normally eat (chips/hotdog/cakes/wine/lager/fattening baguettes). I went to my weigh-in and said to Margaret that I thought I had put on 2 or 3 lb and she said "No you haven't, you've lost one". I need to be good this week as I am sure some of it may catch up with me. I tried to be good today, though we went out. I had an egg mayo sandwich (probably very fattening), and a vanilla milkshake!

Thursday 29th August 2002

An ok day, yesterday R and I went to Southport, got blisters on my feet walking round!!

Went to the Linedancer office where N works and saw Steve as well, R is smitten!

I bought a HUGE jar of sweets the other day (meant to last for AGES) and almost without my knowing I have been raiding the jar all through the day. Food, did I eat food today??? No not really, after all the sweet picking I was not hungry!! Dumb or what!

Friday 30th August 2002

Went to my mum n dads for the day. It is harder to stick to any diet plan when you are out, especially when someone else is doing the cooking. I think I did ok... that is until N came for us and on the way home we called at the Little Chef. I was not in the mood for a meal of any sort... so what did I have??? I shared a huge ice-cream sundae with R and ate some mini donuts and a coffee (all in all about the same amount of cals as a meal, perhaps more?)

Sunday 1st September 2002

Watched a Jason Lee film last night, a romantic comedy. I SOOOOOOOOOOO enjoyed it, plus I fancy Jason Lee like mad!! (God I am getting sad admitting to a film star crush!) Well here's the blurb on the film...

What do you do if you're about to get married and you get cold feet? If you're Max Abbitt (David Schwimmer) you ask your best friend Jay (Jason Lee) to sleep with your fiancee. Max, a sportscaster dedicated to playing the field, and the beautiful intelligent Samantha are a mismatch made in heaven. Jay, who recently had his heartbroken couldn't be unhappier for them. Before he knows it, Max is giving up swinging singlehood but the thought of one woman for the rest of his life suddenly throws Max into a panic. Max reasons that if Samantha cheats on him first, he'll be off the hook. When he asks Jay to help him "test" the relationship, not only does Jay think Max is deranged, but Jay wants nothing to do with the scheme. Unfortunately a little compromising finds Jay and Samantha and Max in an awkward position.

Guess who falls in love with who!!!!!!!!!!!!!!!!!!!!!

Slimming World Week 44

Weight This Week = 9 st 10 lbs (136 lbs)
Loss = 1 lb
Total Lost So Far = 30 lbs

Monday 2nd September 2002

Ok here we go again, another weigh-in day. I feel I ate badly last week. Mainly I have not been bothering to plan or do any cooking so I have just grabbed things as I have gone along.

How did I do it?? How, how?? But I'm glad I did!!! Saw a woman today who I haven't seen for ages and she commented on my weightloss. It is Sooooooooo nice when people notice. Mainly my friends don't cos they see me so often. Steve used the word 'skinny' argghhhhhhhhhh... that is so motivating... I want to be truly skinny. Ok, so I will never be stick thin (wouldn't want to be). Even at my lowest weight of 8 st (112 lbs) you could never say I was thin. I am hoping that by losing another 16 lbs or so I will finally lose my 'stomach'. Yikes... I hope so!!!

Tuesday 3rd September

Judith came round and we went to the park to play tennis with the kids, the balls were flying everywhere!! Grrrrrrrr... we went shopping to Tesco last night, with very few £'s I might add, so no buying junk food. N wanted a small chocolate fix, so I thought Mmmmm I could have one since I lost 1 lb this week (yes... good sensible reasoning). So I had a snickers bar. Bought some cheap chocolate desserts for the kids (I ate just 2 of them). On a roll or what!!!!!!!!!!????? Judith is going to join Slimming World next week (I bet she has a good old 'pig' out the rest of this week. I would!)

Wednesday 4th September

Ha, have been in such a mood today, everything has got on my nerves, just everything. Even eating has gotten on my nerves. I am thoroughly fed up with my stomach (as in the size of it) YUCK it is so there and I want rid of it NOW. Doesn't matter what I wear to disguise it... I know it's there... it's round and too BIG. That's not why I have been in a mood but it has not helped. And it's not PMS (or PMT whatever you call it), it's just plain old being in a bad mood all day!!

Friday 6th September

I bought some chocolate (for the kids - they do so well for chocolate and desserts and things, me being a good mother n all) and have been nibbling it (well eating it in big chunks really). So I had no evening meal (for my penance) - ok, so did not feel like eating cos the chocolate made me sick). So what a waste of calories or what. Why didn't I just have a small amount of choccy and have left it at that - a nice little treat???? No... not me... would I do that?

Sunday 8th September

Arrrrrrrrgh, I don't want to get weighed tomorrow really I don't. Can I stand being told I have gained weight??? My own fault of course - have been eating crappily again all week despite promises to myself that I wouldn't. N did well and is now down to 18 st again (after holiday gain) (that's 252 lbs). I want to make an effort, I want to get my weight going down again. I cannot wait till R goes to school then I can go and do some exercise at the gym (joints allowing of course). I should do some new photos for the photos page (when I am in a less FAT mood).

Slimming World Week 45

Slimming World
Weight = 9 st 12 lbs/138 lbs
Gain = 2 lb
Total Loss = 28 lbs

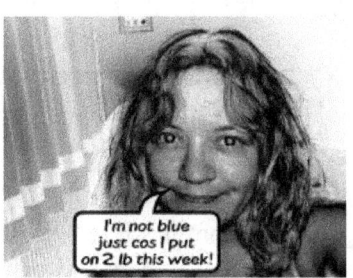

Really honestly it doesn't bother me at all (ermmmm... ok just a bit!)

But who's fault is a weight gain? Can't blame N can I??

Nah!

Monday Sept 2002

Yes here's another weigh-in day and I am hoping for a good weightloss. Ohhh, I am Sooooo not looking forward to getting weighed. I wonder if Judith will come along??

Ok, Ok I put on 2 lb, I knew I had. Judith came along to the meeting (my original diet buddy!!), now she has joined SWorld I bet we are on the phone even MORE!!! After the meeting we went over to the butchers and bought meat (for Red days!) and lots of veg and fruit. I have planned my next 2 days and am going to stick to the plan all week - I will be SO good.

Thursday Sept 2002

STICK TO IT!!!!

Friday Sept 2002

I have not been feeling too well lately, have had major pains in my joints and my blummin blood sugars have been HIGH. I was very lucky to have been given a new machine

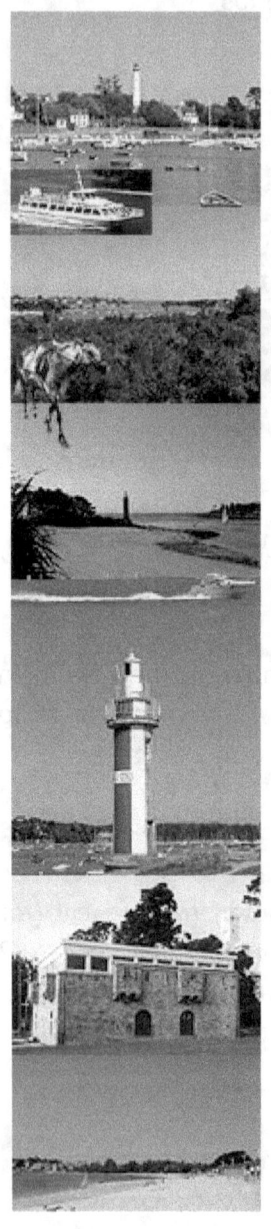

from hubby's boss, it is great and I can painlessly test on my arms (leaving no marks). Can't stop testing... it's fun... though the results aren't. I have actually been eating better this week... writing down everything, counting my 'sins'. Judith came round and helped me prepare my lunch the other day (as I could not cut up the tomatoes or onions). I am determined to lose weight his week. Oh my goodness... I have gone and booked next year's holiday TRULY I have. We are going to a campsite (not the favest of places) but it looks great for the kids, is near a beach and some beautiful places to visit, near enough so N does not have to loads of driving. It is SOOOOO hard finding a holiday to please everyone... next to impossible almost. It is my 40th birthday next year (groan)... but... but... so what, I don't look it so there.

Benodet Images to the left.

We are staying in a campsite called La Pointe St-Gilles, Benodet, France.

I WILL be SOOOOOOOOO slim for this holiday!

Saturday Sept 2002

We went for a walk to the village (a rare thing). Exercise! But on the walk back we had chips off the chippy (also a rare thing!). N and I shared, so I didn't feel half so bad.! I took some photos (or N did) for the site, I was not happy with them, they caught me well... looking FAT and I was NOT in a fat mood, honest.

Sunday Sept 2002

Dunno what to eat today?? N has gone in to work (with Steve...). Being bored makes you want to EAT. I am trying not to.

Slimming World Week 47

Slimming World Weigh-In
Weight =9 st 12 lbs (138 lbs)
Stayed the same
Total Loss So Far = 28 lbs

Monday 16th September 2002

Here we go again, another weigh-in... how have I done?? They are doing a food tasting at SW this week, everyone has to take in some low sin/no sin foods, and just my luck I cannot go... well I can go to get weighed but cannot stay to the meeting cos I have to take R for a hearing test. Never mind. Well I got to the meeting (just), made the 'taster' session. Someone had made simply gorgeous chicken curry (with banana). I stayed the same... I really must try harder this coming week. N is in such a crabby mood (this combined with the kids squabbling makes me want to eat/pick/pig out)

Thursday 19th September 2002

Have had a few bad days where I have eaten crappily, biscuits etc. The kids have started school and they are on packed lunches so there have been more biscuits in the house and of course when I am fed up or whatever, I go have the odd biscuit here and there (too often). I haven't been feeling very well lately, so that doesn't help. I need to think more about what I am eating and get control. I want to get my weight moving again, it does get you down when you have weeks where your weight stays much the same.

Friday 20th September 2002

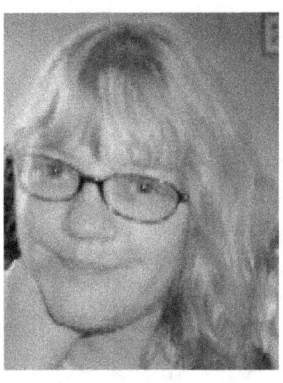

Here I am with my new glasses on, they look bigger than I think they look/seem to be on. I have also got my contact lenses when I want to wear them, but mostly I wear glasses. It is nice to wear the contacts when I go out (on those rare occasions!). I am feeling in a rather FAT mood lately which is getting me down. I bought a pair of size 12 jeans today (beige ones) and they fit me (well I have to lie on the bed to fasten them) and I cannot breathe with them on...but they look good. Now all I need to do is lose another 10 lbs and they will be fine. I though about getting the size 14's but they looked rather big. All my FAT life I have had to wear bigger clothes but when it came to trousers it was a nightmare. My legs have never been fat, I always had skinny legs, so when I had to get say size 18 trousers, they were ridiculously too big in the legs, but fitted on my ermmm big tummy/bum.

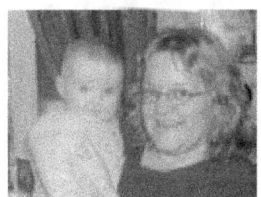

Here I am with my niece in December 2001. I was about 20 lbs heavier here than I am now.

Saturday 21st September 2002

What an awful day, my joints have been hurting so much. I have also eaten SOOOO badly. I need to have myself a good week for once. I did buy loads of fruit yesterday and various other stuff so am armed with the kinda foods I need to stick to the plan.....so...all I need to do now is FOLLOW IT.

Sunday 22nd September 2002

My hands are so bad and I have been feeling so awful. I have eaten so much rubbish, not stuck to the plan at all and even stuffed myself with chocolate today, just felt like it. I cannot undo what I have eaten but I can try and have a better week this coming week, no matter how yuck I feel. Feeling sick is no excuse for overeating, but I am only human!!! I am due to go and see the rheumatology Consultant on the 1st and hopefully they (he) will increase my Methotrexate (am on 12.5mg at moment) and this will sort me out. I also take Vioxx (50-100mg day). I am tired of feeling tired, but I know this is a side effect of the arthritis flare-up. My diabetes is not too bad, am testing regularly (though I know my choccy attack was not a good idea!). I am SOOOOOOOOOO tired all the time, can sleep all day and I mean ALL DAY and still feel tired. I want my energy back. Eating better will help, so this week, tomorrow...I am going to take care of what I eat.

Slimming World Week 47

Slimming World Weigh-In
Weight this week = 9 st 12 lbs
(138 lbs)
STAYED THE SAME
Total Loss so far = 28 lbs

Monday 23rd September 2002

Got weighed and I stayed the same. I am pleased, though I know I have had a bad week last week especially all the chocolate I scoffed yesterday so I simply have to be on the PLAN the whole week this coming week.

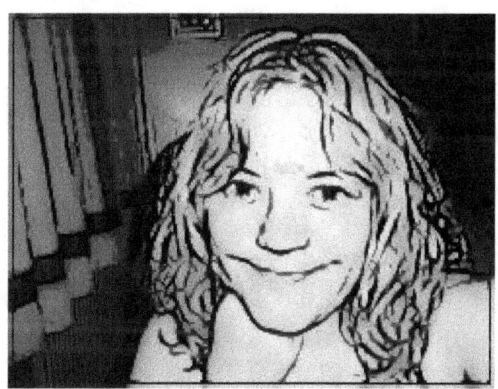

Tuesday 24th September 2002

Have found this great online image changer. It is kodak.com you can upload your digital or scanned images and play around with them, as you can see above/and right, you can cartoon them...also you can order prints and gifts....great fun. Am trying to be good, was not so good last night (it does not help when I feel so YUCK). I ate 2 choccy biscuits/packet of crisps now I have to put these on the days to come as 'sins', that way at least I will be sticking to the plan (in theory!)

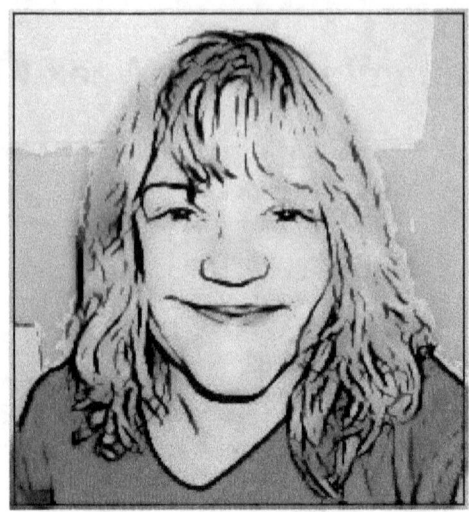

Cartoon me taken 24th Sept 2002

Thursday 26th September 2002

Oh YUCK, I wish I didn't feel so yuck. I feel even yucker cos I stepped on my scales and they say I have gained 2 lb. Of course I have to wait till Mondays weigh-in but I know I JUST KNOW that even if I ate NOTHING till then that I would not lose that 2 lb. Serves me right mind you, I have had a great deal of chocolate oh and a few packets of crisps and the odd biscuit here and there....I have been UN-WELL...really I have. I want to go to the gym, I do, but cannot at the moment. I am hoping to be able to go even if it just means lying on the toning tables to begin with.

Sunday 29th Sept 2002

Took R out yesterday to a 'Fun' day thingy with Kim and Maddy, so Neil got a few hours to himself (hoped this helped?). J was away at Scout camp last night, back today. Yes another week has gone back and still according to my scales I have gained 2 lb and to add to it I feel FAT. Spoke to Judith last night, she has not had a good week either. I have put 70 pennies in a little plastic box and am going to be taking them out as I use them....1 penny per sin. A silly idea perhaps but I am hoping it will help me stick to the plan at least for a time. I have stayed the same weight the last 3 weeks and now a gain (I am sure) and this is well.....stupid. I have been doing so well and I want to get rid of this last 20 lbs and NOT gain any. I know if I don't start eating properly it would be so easy to gain weight. Neil has not been doing well...he has gone back to 18 st 7 lbs, having gained 9 lbs (not in one week). He is very depressed at the moment and fed up (not 100% sure why) and this does not help at all. I want to go back to the gym but my joints are so bad at the moment, though saying that I am going to see the consultant on Tuesday....Once sorted out perhaps I can go to the gym, even if I just go on the toning tables. Kim is wanting to join the gym, this got me to thinking I ought to go. Neil has just told me he has lost 2 lbs this week and now is 18 st 5 lbs!!!!

Slimming World Week 48

Slimming World Weigh-In
Weight this week = 9 st 13 lbs
that's 139 lbs (groan)
Gained 1 lb this week
Total lost so far = 27 lbs

Monday 29th September 2002

Another weigh-in day. Oh I do SOOOOO not want to get weighed today! Ok, ok so I gained a lb. I know why. Now forget it....I am moving on! I am not going to moan groan and beat myself up over it, no, I am just going to do better this week. I have my 70 sins in a little plastic tub (to keep track of... you are allowed 70 'sins' on the Slimming World plan) If you stick to the sins, or have less than you are allowed then you DO lose weight.

Wednesday 2nd October 2002

Went to the Rheumatologist yesterday, they have put up my MTX and I had a steroid jab. I have been counting my sins and taking the pennies out of the tub...so I am pleased about this. When I start feeling better I am definitely going to go to the gym.

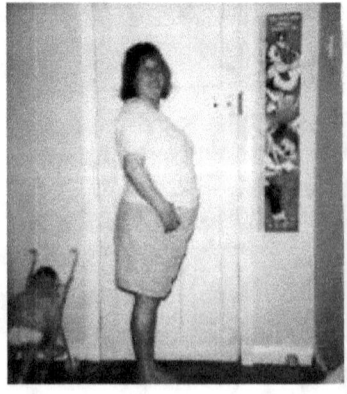 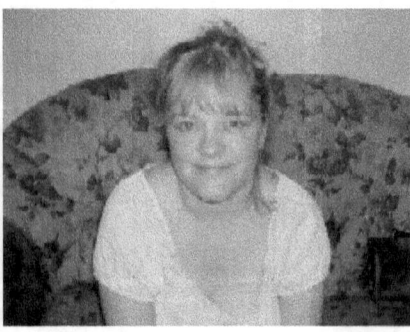

The first picture above was taken around May 2001 I think I weighed 11st 12 lbs (that's 166 lbs) and the 2nd was taken a week ago I was 9 st 12 lbs (that's 138 lbs)

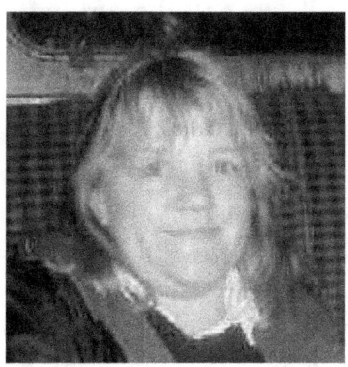

This was me LAST Christmas (Xmas 2001), I had been losing weight and was feeling good about it, but now looking at this photo... It's MEGA MEGA horrid and cringe making, talk about having treble chins! I was 156 lbs

Thursday 3rd October 2002

ARRRGGGGHHHHH........I want chocolate, nothing else will do. I want lots of it. Actually, it's only because we have a load in, lots for J to take on his Scout trip this weekend coming and lots for R's party on the 11th. And because I know it's there in the cupboards, I WANT SOME. It is 20 to 1 in the morning and I have finally come to bed after some riveting episodes of the Outer Limits, I've had 2 cups of coffee/cups of tea/a mug of low fat options drink (2 sins)/some quorn meat (Free and not that fantastic tasting on it's own but what the hell it was food) . I know how easy it would be to RAID the cupboards - why do I torture myself?? But the thing is I know if I do go on a binge I will not lose any weight this week, I have been the same for the last 3 weeks and even gained 1 last week and am MEGA unhappy with my weight still. I know I can successfully lose weight (I have been doing it) - so why continually spoil it?? I can get into smaller clothes this Christmas and not cringe when I see photos, I know I can.

Saturday 5th October 2002

Phew thought I'd lost all the writing off my site, it was not showing up on Dreamweaver at all...HELP....Neil.....HELP. It's ok, sorted out now.

Well......weighed myself on my scales (Yes I know I shouldn't) but they said 9 st 7.5 lbs (131.5 lbs) arhhhhhhhhhh....have not weighed this for years. Ok so SW scales weigh me 2 lb heavier...but I got to almost 9 and a half stones on my scales, it said it there in LCD, in red, stayed there, never budged!!!!! Oh I am feeling so much slimmer. No way hose(a) am I going to sabotage my efforts now and eat junk food (tempting though it is). I want to be under 9 st for Christmas, well as near to 8 st as possible....I want to weigh under 120 lbs (under 8 st 7 lbs) - that is my aim. Now if I went by my scales I am just 16 lbs away from this!!!!!!! That will be my Christmas present to myself.....the weight I want to be, when I get there I can worry about how to stay there!!!!! No NOT YET. I have dug out some more FAT photos of myself and must put them online....to remind me of how I was and how I don't want to look again. I do need to get some exercise though, I have been thinking this. Not easy with the pain I have been in...but it is getting better, I am feeling better so I am going to get doing some exercise. Back to the gym, as I keep saying...I am still paying.

Slimming World Week 49

Slimming World Weigh-In
Weight This Week= 9 st 7 lbs (133 lbs)
Loss= 6 lbs (oh my god!)
Total Loss So Far = 33 lbs

As you can see I have been doing SW for almost 1 year now, whatever is my total loss on week 52...well, I know it will definitely be less than 1 year ago and considering that I have been trying to lose weight since I had R in 1997, I will be very pleased with how I well have done since joining SW. And it does not end there......

ONWARDS and DOWNWARDS

Monday 7th October 2002

Wonder how I will do today?? I don't know how I did it.....I mean yes I stuck to the eating plan, very much so..and I have stayed the same for almost a month (and gained 1 lb) But I have lost 6 lb.......yes a WHOLE 6 pounds since last week. Taking me down to 9 and a half stones (133 lbs). It still hasn't sunk in!! Trouble is I am too scared to eat ANYTHING now (don't wanna gain next week).!! Oh I am sure my appetite will kick in!!!! I have been on the phone ringing up everyone telling them how well I did this week, I kind of ran out of people to phone...and ran out of steam. Neil happened to ring not long after I got home from my meeting and was thrilled. . Everyone's idea of what is overweight or not is totally different. I have very skinny friends who moan about being 'fat'. AIMed (like Instant messenger) Steve and I think he was quite amazed!!!

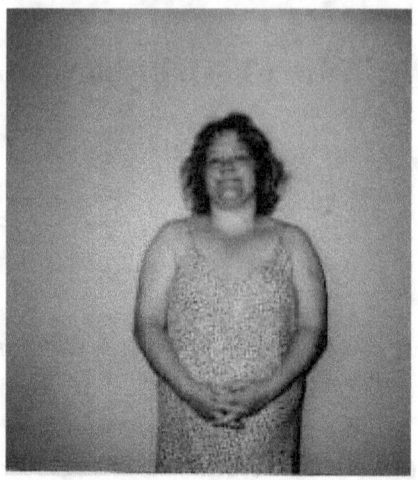

Here I am I think it was Summer 2001, I remember getting this dress and thinking I looked slim in it....I don't think so! (I think I was about 11 st 5 lbs or 161 lbs)

I think I will have to take more photos tonight and put them up - so you can see the difference more.

Tuesday 8th October 2002

Ok day. Have not eaten too much so far! Rang Judith, she is doing ok too and said she is in a cooking mood. I have got to help Neil get back on track, he has not been doing so well lately, he has gone back to snacking at night, which is fine if you don't overdo it. It is hard cos he has such a big appetite, though he was gaining control of it and starting to feel better.

Friday 11th October 2002

Arghhhhhhh, did R's party today. It was knackering, but lovely. It is her 5th birthday tomorrow/ She had lots of lovely girly pressies. I managed to eat a few pieces of cake and ok a few chocolaty nibbles here and there (I was stressed! and tempted)

Saturday 12th October 2002

R's 5th Birthday. Most of my family came round with presents. More cake to hand out and more to tempt me! So of course I know who to blame for me putting on weight this week (ME).

A sweet Little Girl is 5

Sunday 13th Oct 2002

Neil has lost 2 lbs this week, taking him down to 18 st 3 lbs (255 lbs). I dared to step on my scales and have weighed the same (clothes off though!). Have counted out my pennies for the week and I am going to stick to the plan....

I SOOOOOOOOOOOOOOOOO want to lose the last of my weight for Christmas, which is (counting tomorrow) 10 weigh-ins away, this takes me up to my last weigh in before Christmas on the 23rd December. Depending on how my joints are this week I am going to go along to the gym.

Slimming World Week 50

Slimming World Weigh-In
Weight = 9 st 7 lbs (133 lbs)
Loss/Gain =SAME
Total Lost So Far = 33 lbs

Monday 14th October 2002

I am sure I have gained some weight this week....almost CERTAIN I have. We shall see. But with losing the 6 lbs last week and R's birthday just gone (and I had a few pieces of cake and a few other nibbles!!)

Phew!!!!! I have stayed the same weight this week. That is great, I really thought I might have a gain, but haven't....now am determined to push on for next week, I want to lose 2 lb for next week. Judith came round for a coffee, she has stayed the same this week (and had her birthday!!)

Wednesday 16th October 2002

Went to Heswall this morning for a wander. Saw a few people who said they didn't recognise me...oh REALLY? I don't think I have changed THAT much, made me feel brill though.....it is so nice when people see that I have lost weight (as opposed to my family who say nothing much although they ought to be forgiven since they see me fairly oftenish) I have been quite desperate for salted peanuts (Judith says I must need the salt since we have none in the house - I never ever use it). I had to buy some s. peanuts for the meeting tonight (at the hospital with the consultants - a nibbles affair - I am in charge of some nibbles!) I have had ok a few handfuls of peanuts...just a few and have had to put them AWAY for fear of eating them ALL!!!!!!

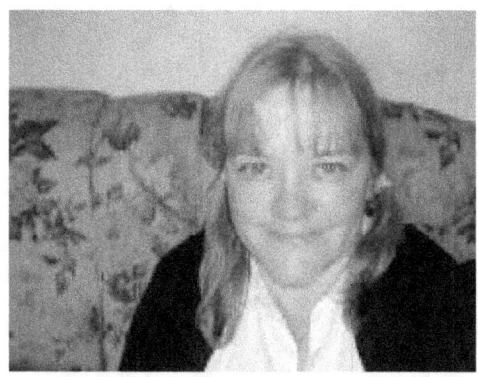

Naff hairstyle I know (am about 30 years too old for bunches but SO WHAT)(photo taken today by me with the digital camera at arms length!!........OK so I am a BIT vain!)

Thursday 17th October 2002

Am going to see Swan Lake (with Moscow Ballet Company) next week at the Liverpool Empire Theatre with my friend Nicola (it's her birthday). Am really looking forward to it. Does everyone get dressed up? The kids are off school next week (half term hols) so.....activities??? Bread making (as promised), maybe a train ride?? Visits to friends houses? Arghhhhhh toothache. Why me. One thing, it stops you from eating so much, last 2 nights, no nibbling, no snacking just a few painkillers and bed. What a pain.

Saturday 19th October 2002

Went to the dentist yesterday, was given antibiotics. Toothache is just loathsome really painful and it kept me awake all last night, despite bucketfuls of painkillers. It is non stop pain that you can't get away from. It's not like I don't visit the dentist regularly....some people have problems with their teeth and I'm one of them at the moment. I think Neil is a saint for putting up with my wailing. Is it time for more painkillers, I know you should be careful but they way it hurts I don't care at the moment. Dentist sent me away to come back on the 11th YES the 11th November (waiting for antibiotics to work I presume, that and 'Peter' is on holiday)....god can I wait that long???? Can Neil put up with me that long? Can I put up with me that long? Toothache is so trivial, not like some awful disease, but it HURTS Soooooooooooo much.

Slimming World Week 51

Slimming World Weigh-In
Weight = 9 st 5 lbs (131 lbs)
Loss = 2 lbs
Total Lost = 35 lbs

Monday 21st October 2002

Well, how will I do today?? Ok I hope! I stepped on my scales Saturday morning and they said 9 st 4 lbs? Wonder how they will compare to SW?? Should ONLY go by SW scales but it is so tempting to step on my scales. Neil stayed the same this week. Can you believe it I lost another 2 lbs! I got my one and a half stone sticker today. I ran into the meeting (normally I always stay but couldn't cos I had to go to the dentist), but I was determined to go and get weighed. I am only about 12 lbs away from the weight I want to be. (Of course I may go for weighing even less but, we shall see). I have had stronger painkillers from the dentist so I HOPE these get to work.

Tuesday 22nd October 2002

Well I am soon off to the Ballet (To see Swan Lake in Liverpool Empire - Moscow Ballet Comp) And wouldn't you know it...it's a FAT day. Yesterday wasn't, not the day before not the day before that, but today is an I feel FAT/HUGE/NOTHING FITS day. Had my outfit hanging up for the last week or so, fitted lovely, room to breath and...and...get my hand down my pants (sorry not being rude here) now I am wondering how do I go to the loo in the theatre and fasten my trousers without lying on the floor???????? Where did that BIG stomach come from?? Ok so it's a fair way to go but it was deflating, it was, but suddenly it's popped out (up?) again. Was it those crisps I ate yesterday?? Is my body getting me back for eating (pigging out on) ermmmm.....4 or so packets of them (I loathe to mention this).

It's not fair

Wednesday 23rd Oct 2002

The Ballet (English Ballet Company it was) was WONDERFUL and beautiful. I was torn though between wanting to watch the ballet and the orchestra - the music/musicians were very impressive. The theatre was packed, we had good seats. I can't think why I have never been to such a performance (or to the theatre in general) before, it is soooooo nice.

Today I went to the dentist again, she took another x-ray. Ah she could see the infection more (like I never knew I had it!) And I am having the tooth removed tomorrow. I feel sick at the thought....but I know it is for the best. I am so tired of the pain. I've eaten badly but then perhaps I am forgiven for this week?

Thursday 24th Oct 2002

Had my tooth out, it was not as bad as I thought it would be. Now I am wondering what I can eat? Hah typical!! No way will I have a weightloss this week.

Friday 25th October 2002

Have been eating all comfort foods now I can!!! Will have to make an effort to stop before it becomes a massive binge. It can be so easy to go off track. Nicola came round and she looked after the kids while I went to the dentist (yes again) and I bought her a little bag of choccies as a thank you...of course I tried one or two.

Saturday 26th Oct 2002

I cannot believe all the extra stuff I have been eating.....even with all the pain of toothache and having the tooth out. Chocolate, the 2 cakes I ate the other night as a treat for having tooth out, the Mars Bar I had today cos I was out shopping and in a rush, the garlic bread I had the other night cos I had MAJOR toothache and was hungry, the chocolate fingers I sucked at the beginning of the week cos I could not chew..............etc etc. And my scales say I have gained at least 3 lbs and I know, lets have a Chinese takeaway tonight (cos I can just about chew now and deserve a treat) and add a few more lbs to my body. How can 1, just 1 tooth lead to this????????????????????

Slimming World Week 52

MY Weight After 1 year at Slimming World
Weight = 9st 6 lbs (132 lbs)
Gain = 1 lb
Total Lost So Far = 34 lbs

It is one year since I started Slimming World and as you can see I HAVE FINALLY LOST WEIGHT (ok more to lose but...) I am really pleased with how I have done and I promise myself I will not let the odd gain here and there undo all the weight I have lost.

Monday 28th October 2002

Can you believe I went to the gym yesterday, I only stayed an hour but at least I went!!! I am going to try and go more often to make up for the last weeks binging and to help get rid of this last 14 or so lbs.

I wonder how I have done this week?? I know I must have gained weight cos of all the binging I did last week....but This is Week 52, so I have been doing Slimming World for ONE YEAR, a whole year ago I was 34 lbs heavier! One year ago I weighed 11 st 12 lbs (166 lbs) . As you can see I gained a pound, which is ok since I ate so badly last week. I went to the gym after slimming world - aren't I good!!!!!

Tuesday 29th October

I was doing so well yesterday really I was. Then I opened some mint chocolate biscuits and JUST had to have one....but did I have one???? No I only went and had 6....yes 6, that's a whole/whopping 27 sins in one go. But...but I counted them, so I have less room for treats for the rest of the week...but serves me right!!! I am going to go to the gym later for a hour and burn some calories off on the treadmill. I really want to lose at least 2 lb for next week. Going to the gym is quite addictive, though I do have to be careful (with having the arthritis), I get annoyed that I cannot use all the machines...but I just can't so that's that. Should I have a fitness assessment?? Nah not yet!

Wednesday 30th October

Tonight we (me and J) are going to McDonalds Halloween Party, ok it's for the kids but it is my chance to dress up too, after all parents have to make a bit of an effort! I have won a long red velvet dress off EBay and have paid for it already so I HOPE it gets to me by Wednesday, though I have a horrid feeling it won't. It is a size 16 (12 in the USA), I am now fitting into size 12's (8's on the USA I think?) Anyway, J is going as....dunno.....bloody t-shirt, raggy/slashed trousers - gory. Nicola and her daughter are going as is Judith and her kids....wonder if I'll be the only one dressed up????

Thursday 31st October

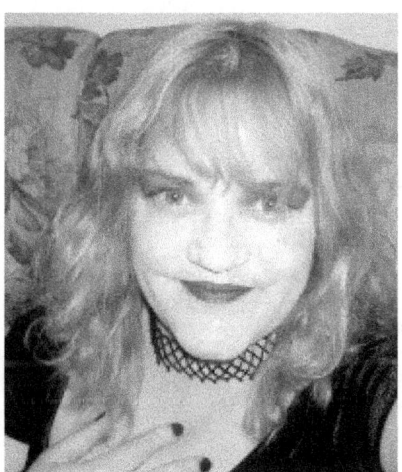

Well, we went to McDonalds and I only had 1 Mcflurry, a plain burger and a small cone, not too bad?? It is very difficult not to eat when everyone else is stuffing themselves!!!! I have been to the gym 3 times in a row so this will help a little bit to cancel out some of the calories I hope!!!

Saturday 2nd November

We are off to my sister-in-laws tonight, nephews 12th birthday/firework party. She will have loads of stuff out and I will be tempted to EAT. So far today I have had fruit and yoghurt for brekky and sandwich for lunch...so my aim is not to eat till tonight?! Why is it when I am trying my best to lose weight, food gets in the way??? Ah yesterday I did my first day at the shop....I am going to do one day a week in Oxfam (on the till), not the most glamorous of jobs (and unpaid) but I hope it will give me some confidence and well....something to put on my c.v since it is so long since I have worked. I will also be helping out in the school on Monday afternoons, then the gym Tuesdays/Wednesdays and Thursdays with the odd weekend stint thrown in...all helps cut down on the time you can eat (can't eat!!!) Pity!!!!

Slimming World Week 53

Slimming World Weigh-In
Weight = 9 st 5 lbs (131 lbs)
Loss = 1 lb (yippee)
Total Lost So Far = 35 lbs

Monday 4th November 2002

I have a secret desire!!!! A silly one really but something I have wanted to do for some time. Don't know if I could afford it or where I could get it done. It would be for me only (ok and Neil) and it might sound like a silly thing....but still. When I have lost all my weight I would love to have a make-over....a 40's makeover - make-up, clothes and hairstyle. Neil says he prefers the 20's look, which is nice I agree, we have some art deco stuff in the house and I have this wonderful photo of my auntie that was taken around 1933 (it was originally a postcard and I got it when she died), I had the postcard made into a larger photograph (cost me £100, she looks beautiful on it, in fact I would love to have it made into a VERY LARGE painting, but the cost would be horrendous). I wonder where in this country you might be able to get such a makeover - the 40's style????

Yeah...I lost the lb I put on last week....now...lets get going DOWN again!!! I want to be Soooooo good this week....starting NOW. I am not going to let crappy eating ruin my goal

Tuesday 5th November 2002

Had a good day today....as in I didn't overdo the crappy eating. J came home with loads of chocolate and I ate some but I counted it. Obviously when you count your 'sins' properly you DO lose weight. I feel Soooooooooo much slimmer (but not on a FAT day). Today was an I feel slim day which is good. Unfortunately it was also an *I have spots* day (arghhhhhhh), as usual on my nose....unhideable, uncoverable very THERE. Well on the 5th of November last year I weighed 11 st 12 lbs (166 lbs), it was my 1st meeting at Slimming World (A Monday Evening) and here I am now at 9 st 5 lbs (131 lbs).

Some days I see myself as still VERY FAT and other days I see myself as almost SKINNY.............it's weird!

Thursday 7th November 2002

I am not very good at drawing, though in my mind I am...funny how you can visualise just how you will draw/paint something then it never comes out like that on paper!! In my minds eye I am brilliant at drawing (NOT!). But I did do the drawing below, using J's school pens! Then I scanned and reduced the size of it...not too bad is it?! I think I was thinking of CHOCOLATE at the time!!!

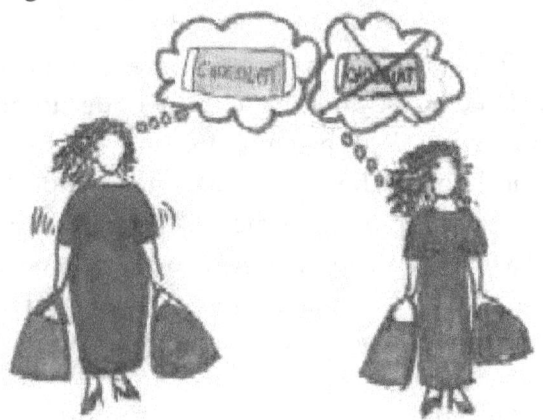

Friday 8th November 2002

Worked in the shop today and really enjoyed it, and managed to do the till right this time!!!! Kim came round and we got all the clothes outta my wardrobe, tried this and that on...not a bad feat considering she is about a foot taller than me! Will I stop having FAT feeling days when I have lost all my weight??? This year I am going (so far) to 3 Christmas party do's (alone) and I am wanting something nice to wear (that makes me look almost thin - is this possible?) At least I will look better than last Christmas...I shall have to dig out that old photo for comparison.

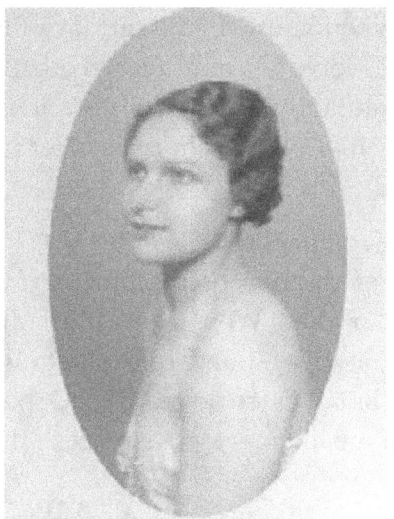

Here is the photo of my Aunty Nellie, I have it in a frame on the wall, one day I am going to afford to get it made into a large painting.

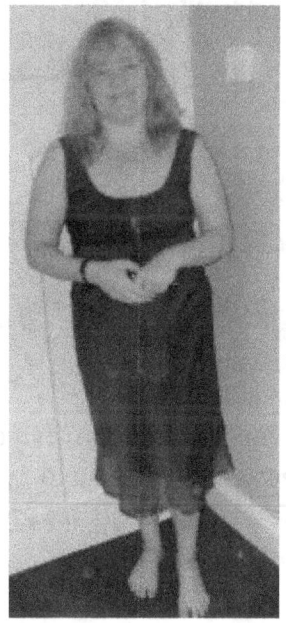

I got this dress to try on (thinking it would look lovely on) but although I love the dress it does not suit me and I felt really FAT in it. I am pleased that it was a 14 and fairly loose, but you know when you get an item of clothing and you are convinced it will look fab and everything.....well....My arms are too fat and so is my face and all of me is still far too fat (moan..moan) AND AND I want to be taller (maybe I ought to buy some shoes?)

Saturday 9th November 2002

Slept most of the day (joints hurting me) which works wonders for your diet. Won a beautiful dress on EBay...a 1950's gown. I know I will never be able to wear it anywhere (unfortunately) but it is so lovely. I DO hope it fits. A bit frivolous (sp?)of me I know. Here is a pic of the dress.

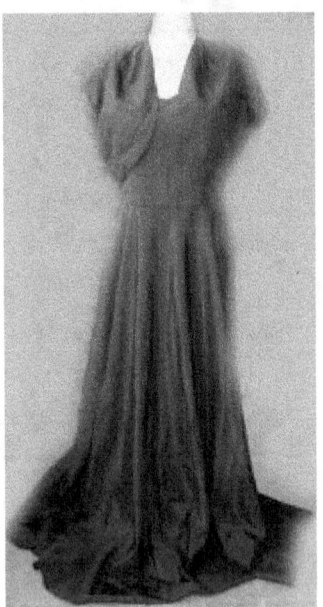

Now.....if it fits me when it arrives you shall see a photo of me in it. Yes..I know it will be too long (what do I expect at only 5 ft). Its is a size 14 (10 USA)(I am getting into these. Oh I know in my mind I am a foot taller but......I can dream.

Sunday 10th November 2002

I am not looking forward to getting weighed tomorrow, I know I have not been trying too hard to follow the Slimming World Plan this last week. I have been getting a bit lazy about it and having foods here and there (picking basically) and saying to myself "Oh this little bit won't matter, I'll count it later" I guess we all get weeks like this but it would be a shame to carry on like this when I am so close to my target. I don't want to be this weight by Christmas.

Slimming World Week 54

Slimming World Weigh-In
Weight = 9 st 5 lbs (131 lbs)
Stayed the same
Total Lost So Far = 35 lbs

Monday 11th Nov 2002

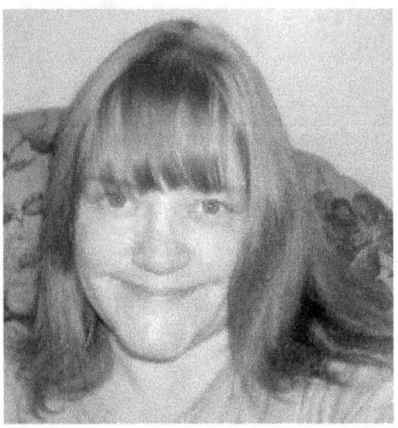

I really don't think I will have lost weight this week, I have not followed the plan as much as I would have liked. So here I am...and I stayed the same which is good, I really must make more of an effort this week. Went to the dentist then bought myself a ham/cream cheese baguette (what was I saying?). And I will count it honestly I will. As you can see here I have coloured my hair today, I like to do this from time to time as I do get bored with it. I do think about having it cut short but on the other hand I love longer hair. I know Neil will say he prefers my hair light blonde!!!

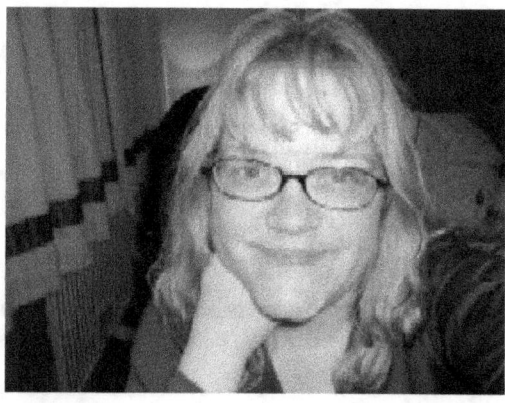

This was taken last week sometime. I am so vain I know! Part of me wants to keep taking photos cos I never like how I look in them, I want to look thinner/pretty for once/not so old/have a less chubby face etc etc. I think I always look kind of dumb in my photos, I try to change the way I smile, but I always smile the same way, always.

Tuesday 12th Nov 2002

The ball gown came....it is beautiful, but I need less ermmmm....padding (me) around the ribs!! I am hoping when I lose the rest of my weight it will at least zip up! I also bought a new coat today (a size 14) and it fits beautifully, I am really pleased with it. I think back to last year when even a size 18 would have been too tight......it is still weird getting into smaller sizes. I have eaten ok today...as in I have not picked... this helps when you have very little in the kitchen cupboards!!

Wednesday 13th Nov 2002

The Ball gown fits.. it fits... it really fits. When I got up this morning (as you do), I hopped out of bed and since I was ermmm...naked and Neil was around (god this sounds awful)...I decided to put the dress on just to show him how much it did not fit. I said "Can you zip it up for me?" thinking he might at least be able to zip it part way and Lo and Behold it zipped all the way up...without me having to breathe in. It must have been the angle I was at that made it next to impossible for me to zip it up. I was Soooooooooooooooo pleased. Got Neil to take some photos of me in it (yes at 7.30 in the morning), but was not to pleased with how I looked in the photos (knackered). So when I get some decent photos in the next day or so I will put them on the site. I was aiming to be good today but I went and bought some chocolate from the shop (for the kids) and then I got a bit stressed out later on and ate a fair bit of it. Why oh why is it so easy to go and eat all the wrong things, why oh why do I head for the kitchen when I feel even the tiniest bit fed up/stressed/bored/down etc???????

Thursday 14th Nov 2002

Went shopping to Cheshire Oaks and bought a few Christmas presents (just a few). When I am the weight I want to be I am going to go to lots of shops and try stuff on (maybe).

Inside me there's a thin person struggling to get out, but I can usually sedate her with four or five cupcakes.

Friday 15th Nov 2002

Blummin BT... have not been able to upload my site for ages, they were supposed to sort it out... yeah like WHEN?.

Saturday 16th Nov 2002

Didn't do very much today, though did manage to go in a shop and get some sweeties and eat them...toffees no less.. I don't want to have put weight on when I go on Monday, I really don't. I know I have gradually gotten worse over the week and eaten more fattening stuff... the same old thing saying to myself "Oh I'll count that tomorrow" and then I don't count that tomorrow.

Sunday 17th Nov 2002

Well my scales say I have lost a bit....but I will have to wait till the morning to see. Neil and I went shopping and I got an urge for curly wurlys and bought a pack of 5, trouble is I ate 4 of them (WHY?). I have my chocolate urges again.....grrrrrrrrrrrrrr. Inbetween this and that I am eating properly of course! There are 5 weigh-ins till Christmas (this takes me up to the last weigh in before Xmas on the 23rd December). If I lost say 2 lb tomorrow (that's take me to 9 st 3 or 129 lbs) then I lost just over 2 lb a week till Xmas then THEN I would get to my GOAL weight on the 23rd December. But we all know how in the past I have said (if I lose this by......" and I HAVEN'T)...so, whatever...I will be very pleased to lose some weight or even stay the same. I must try and stick to my Slimming World Plan and have the correct amount of sins and I know I will do well, I have proved this to myself by losing all the weight I have done so far. My biggest breakthrough will be when I get under 9 st (and be 8 st something), that's under 126 lbs. I have not been under this weight for over 10 years. When I first met Neil I was 112 lbs (8 st) and I covered up cos I felt fat, how silly. I remember going to bed (when I first ermmm did with Neil) with more clothes on than I wore in the day including socks and I did this for ages!!! I never wore anything tucked in (stomach too big.....not!!!!). When I went out to pubs/discos with my sisters or friends, they wore next to nothing (mum complained "you'll freeze to death")..she never had to say that to me!!!!!

Perhaps now after being overweight I will appreciate being slimmer, I will feel better about my body....I won't feel constantly fat anymore??? Till the next time I wake up in the morning and it's a FAT day of course.

Yes ONLY 35 days to Christmas!!

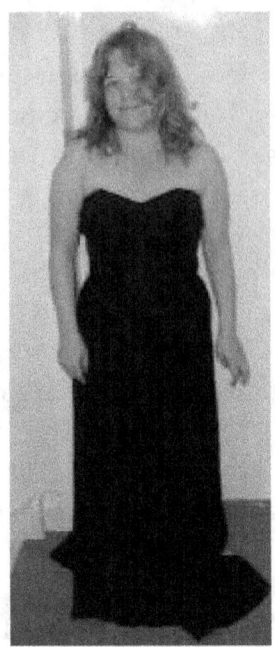

Here I am in the Ball gown I bought recently, not the best photo (7am in the morning and uncombed hair!) But like I said I got the gown on.....Last Christmas it would not have gone near me.

Slimming World Weigh-In

(Monday 18th November 2002)

Weight this week = 9st 4 lbs (130 lbs)
Loss = 1 lb
Total Lost So Far = 36 lbs

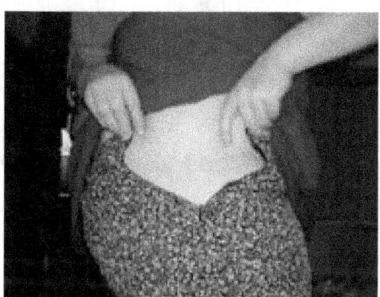

11th Feb 2002
10st 12 lbs (152 lbs)

A very long way from fastening here.
(My stomach is on the left!)

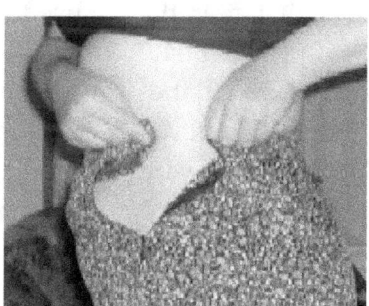

9th Aug 2002
9st 11 lbs (137 lbs)
Getting closer, the top of the zip nearly meets.

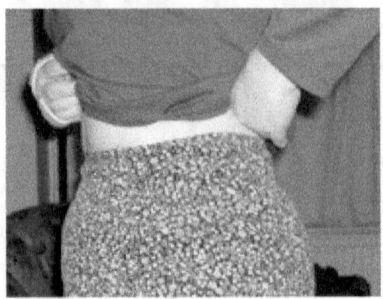

15th Nov 2002
9 st 5 lbs (131 lbs)

Only 6 lbs difference from when I last tried the skirt on...but now it fastens easily, although I have not lost that many pounds perhaps my body shape has changed and I have lost more inches off my waist.

Monday 18th November 2002

I wonder how I will do today?? I hope I have lost some. Well I lost another pound, this is great. I am just 11 lbs away from my target. I still find it hard to believe that I have lost all this weight after trying on and off for years to lose weight and never getting anywhere. I eat far better than I ever have, ok so I have the odd binge and still eat junk food here and there but somehow I do it all better than I used to...I have a better balance. Did I really eat SO badly in the past, obviously I did, hence the weight gain ad the trouble getting any off. The beauty of the Slimming World plan is that I can stay on it forever...it is such a healthy way of eating and is well.....normal and not faddy. I don't let food rule my life, I accept the odd gain here and there and I definitely don't deny myself all the things I like. I do eat out less and have much fewer takeaways (which were always highly fattening), they are nice for the odd treat, but in the past it was more than the odd treat it was almost weekly!

Tuesday 19th November 2002

Have eaten very little today, not that hungry. Though saying that I did overdo the chocolate yesterday so perhaps it's just as well. I was saying to my Slimming World Consultant Carole how I find it difficult sometimes to go for smaller sizes in the shops. I find myself being very reluctant to get size 14's(10 in the USA)(which I can easily get into really - the odd few I have or have tried on). I would never purchase a 12(8 in the USA). Perhaps when I lose this last amount of weight I will feel able to just go and buy then no problem!

Thursday 21st November 2002

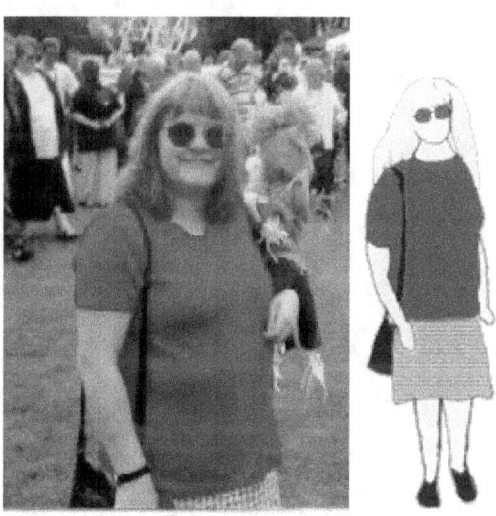

Had a go at drawing myself (sort of!) Hehe. I have been doing a few drawings (by hand, put them up on my drawings page) and I am not very good at it, but perhaps with practise they might get better (or I could trace?). I do like drawing but I am no good at perspective or getting the shape of things right or shadow...or anything like that. If you compared my go at drawing to say J's (my son's who is 11 or even my 5 yr olds!) you might be hard pressed to say who drew what!! I have not been eating properly, sort of skipping meals and not bothering as such. I went to Southport yesterday shopping and went to this coffee shop (Costa) and had the BIGGEST mug (it had 2 handles)of amaretto coffee you have ever seen (thought I'd just try it). The cream on top...well it took me so long to get through it that the coffee was cold when I got to that so I had to ask for a top up of hot water. It was lovely and sickly at the same time!

Sunday 24th November 2002

Went to see Harry Potter Chamber Of Secrets yesterday, I really enjoyed it, so did J. Once again I have exceeded myself in NOT sticking to my 'sins' this last week...hence I expect I shall have a weight gain tomorrow. I am not eating properly, I know this. I am eating the wrong foods and none of the correct ones. It's almost like I can't be bothered??? I must try harder and get back to sensible eating. Made a chicken soup for tomorrow (that's a start!)

Slimming World Week 56

Slimming World Weigh-In
Weight This Week = 9 st 2 lbs (128 lbs)
Loss = 2 lbs
Total Lost So Far = 38 lbs
Number of lbs left to lose = 9 lbs

Things that I do a bit differently now

1. I think about food less and less, mainly only right before it's time to eat (not inbetween)
2. I don't always say YES to that offer of a sweet or nibble etc. (You can say no quite easily...but if you really really want that nibble/snack/chocolate then have it...but don't then go on a binge)
3. I don't buy 'diet food' anymore (I used to spend loads on so called diet foods especially the ermm cake sort, but now I don't bother)
4. I eat more fruit, more so at breakfast.

Monday 25th November 2002

I wonder how I will do today... I always ask this!! I am hoping that at the worst I have stayed the same

I have lost another 2 lbs this week. I WILL have to be better this week, I have not been eating properly....but perhaps not as bad as I thought?? The end is in sight!!! If anyone has said to me a year ago "OH Cathy, it will take at least a year for you to lose your weight".....well I would have given up before I started really I would. The thing this time is I have stuck at it, even when I have put weight on. I know that I have been so much better this last year with my food/eating. I can't say I have exercised that much (I intend to do more exercise).

Wednesday 27th November 2002

I went to a Hotpot Supper last night (with the people I work with at the shop on Fridays)....one of the ladies houses. We had an absolutely delicious Lamb hotpot (stew) and then I had a portion of homemade apricot pie with cream (ok so I should've left out the cream!)....it was so YUMMY. Other people were drinking mulled wine, but I had water or homemade lemonade. I wore a long red velvet dress and a red sparkly bobble in my hair (it is a Christmas 'do'). I felt so much slimmer than I have done for years and for once felt really good about how I looked.

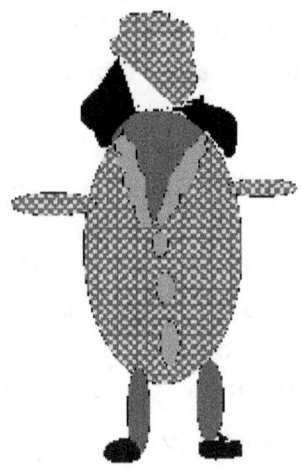

I am not an apple shape
I am not a pear shape
I rather think I am a bit OVAL shaped!

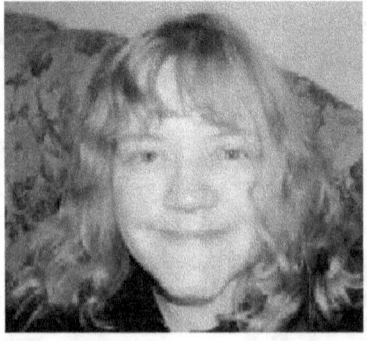

Thursday 28th November 2002

Went shopping and managed to spend very little, but Kim persuaded me to go into Burger King as it was lunch time and we were both hungry. What a waste of calories. I had a chicken burger and fries and coffee and felt yuck after it. Now I wonder how much weight I will have put on this week. I ate badly yesterday. R and I opened a box of After Eight Mints (ok she's 5 and I opened them). We worked our way though almost the whole box (yes I had the most). We did save some for Neil when he got home, though not many. It is awful when I get towards the end of a week and I know I most probably will have gained....you can't turn back the clock. We all have lapses, but sort of doing it each day is a bit too much! Old habits die hard.

I have hopped on my scales (as per usual) and seem to have s small gain (I say this...small....cos it makes me feel better about it). I am hoping that by Monday morning I have lost that small gain and at least stayed the same. But who knows with the human body???? Especially mine. There are chocolate biscuits in the cupboard and I want some...just a few, but over the last week I have my fair share of chocolate really I have.

Sunday 1st December 2002

Went to my parents house yesterday. Spent a few hours in my sister house, she is also following SW, so I managed to eat ok!!! Ermmm...oopps raided her biscuit tin, had a few (say about 6) mini chocolate biccy shapes) arrrggghhhh. Then over at my mums dad had some whisky filled chocolates over from his birthday and I had ohhhhhhhhh 5 of those. It is so easy to forget about these things!!! Other than that I followed the plan.!!!!!!! I know, I just know I will have a little gain this week, I had my mother-in-laws party last Sunday, my hotpot supper on the Tuesday night and my burger king stop off on Wednesday or thereabouts.......plus my other picking (which I am trying to get back out of the habit of doing). But...even with a gain, I will aim to have a better week next week. In the past a small gain would leave me feeling down for ages and make me comfort eat really it would, which is why I never lost any weight. But this time I accept that I am only human and that for the main, I have done well with my weightloss and NO WAY am I going to let it pile back on.

Slimming World Week 57

Slimming World Weigh-In
Weight this week = 9 st 2 lbs(128 lbs)
Stayed the same
Total Lost So Far = 38 lbs
Total left to lose = 9 lbs

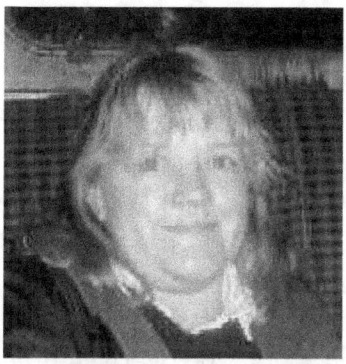

Me last Christmas 2001(the beginning of December)

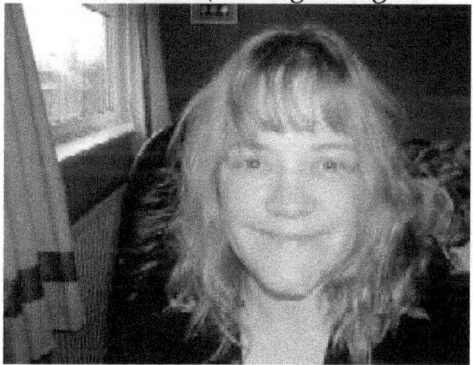

Taken today 2nd December 2002

I remember having the photo taken, the one above. We were out on a day trip to Llangollen to see the Santa Express, me Neil and the kids. I thought I looked ok...well....I had started Slimming World and had lost a few lbs. But when I saw the photo I was horrified at how gross I looked, how fat I looked. When I was overweight I never liked having a BIG round face (not to mention a ermmm...big round body to go with it. J did say to his teacher once that Mummy is a round ball (he was only 5 or 6), now he's 11 and is taller than me and weighs more than me!!

Monday 2nd December 2002

I cannot believe how close we are getting to Christmas. I have done a little bit of shopping so far.

Now....I wonder how my weightloss will be this week....????

Can you believe it... I stayed the same. I was so relieved. I could not stay to the meeting cos J is off sick, it looked like it was going to be a good meeting too. Each time we lose weight we get a gift tag with our name on and these go into a draw. I am going to really stick to the plan this week, I want to be in the 8 stones for Christmas (that's another 4 lb + to lose to be 8 st something). I feel that this nitime, the weight I have lost will stay off and as long as I keep a check on it and don't pile on too many lbs, then I won't be overweight ever again. The last time I was 'slim' was when I met Neil, I weighed 8 st (112 lbs). Unfortunately, as I've said before, I always thought I was overweight even at that weight. My family do have a phobia of weight, I know at various times my sisters have put on a few lbs and it has been terrible for them, Though perhaps in one way this is not too bad, since, if I had tackled my weight when I was just a bit overweight I might never have gotten SO overweight. But this is all 'after the fact'. I got overweight for a variety of reasons (blame hubby and marriage! blame pregnancy etc) and it has taken me 10 years to get slimmer. When I used to catch glimpses of myself in shop windows or even worse shop mirrors, I hated it, all I saw was this fat frumpy person. Now it doesn't bother me - seeing myself. Oh ok I have a groan at say, my knackered looking face (the shop lights are so harsh!), but I am happy at last with how my body looks. Getting down to the nitty gritty, I do need to lose the last of this weight (either that or have surgery on the last of my stomach which still can ermmm......make a slappy noise YUCKEEE when I run down the stairs. There are holderinnerknickers of course but I am hoping when I lose this last 9 lbs or more....that stubborn bit of stomach will disappear!!!! Watch this space!!

Tuesday 3rd December 2002

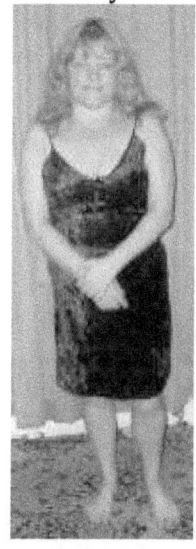

I bought a few dresses today and tried them on and I look huge in them really I do. I cannot wear them, no way. I didn't realise just how BIG I still look in certain things. Take for example this purple dress. I look absolutely dreadful in it. I could not wear this in a million years, it does nothing for me and I do not know why I bought it. In fact I bought another one in grey, a longer one in gold and one in black.....how stupid. I cannot believe I even considered that these dresses might look ok on me. I still have weight to lose, so perhaps I should wait till I get there before I go buy anymore things? The one thing is that these dresses were in the sale and cost very little (thank goodness).

Oh and just for good measure...what have I done this last 2 days??? Overeaten of course. Stuffed my face with chocolate and crisps. We ate out a few times today (cos we were out shopping and treated ourselves), me and Neil this is. SO now I have NO sins left for the week if I want to stand any chance of staying the same. Ok....I will aim to do this. Perhaps I feel particularly fat at the moment cos I have eaten so much lately and it's almost that time of the month???? I thought I was done with feeling like a huge blob...but I'm not. Maybe I ought to choose my clothes more carefully??

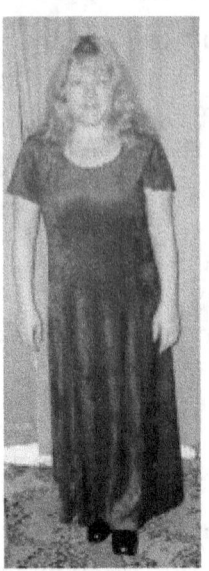

Here is the dress I wore to the Hotpot Supper last week. I must admit looking at a photo of me in it makes me feel I looked fat. Yes, that word again.

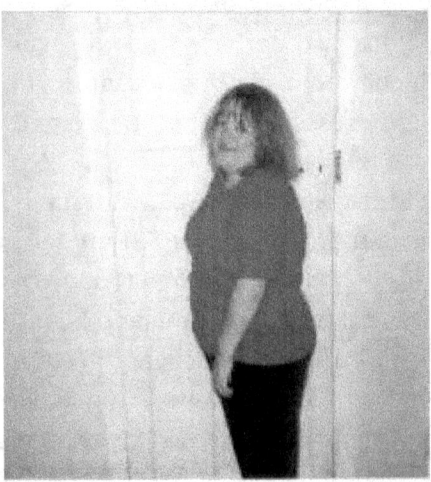

I mean I know I look better now than I did say here in this photo taken when I was about 11 st 7 lbs (161 lbs), but I still feel fat and it's not fair.

Thursday 5th December 2002

I made a teabread and a marmalade cake for the school fair...+ 1 extra teabread (just to test it was ok). I have eaten quite a few pieces, does taste lovely especially with butter on. All I can say is I will certainly not have lost weight this coming Monday but I must do my best not to have any more 'binges'...let's limit the damage shall we.

Saturday 7th December 2002

Am trying very very hard not to get into the festive mood (eating wise!) yet. My 'brain' is telling me 'oooohhhhhh there's some lovely chocolately goodies out there.....lindt and all that'. Oh and it is Christmas (almost) and it is OK to eat all these goodies at Christmas and mince pies and all that.

BUT

I do not want to pile on the lbs right this minute. I am already stressing how FAT I feel and feel I look. We have our Slimming World Christmas Party on Monday night and I have bought a top (the sort that hides your spare tyres but shows a bit of cleavage!!)....now do I wear the black trousers or the long satin skirt??? How very FAT will I feel on Monday??? Of course it depends on HOW much weight I will have gained all this early festive eating.

Sunday 8th December 2002

Went to my mum n dads house. My dad is going into hospital for a double heart by pass operation on Monday (op on Tuesday). He is 58. I think both mum and dad are nervous. Here's a pic of mum and dad last Christmas.

Went over to my sisters who lives over the road from mum n dad, she is following SW diet too, unfortunately she had some Christmassy sweets out and we both indulged. Today is the last day or overindulging, I have had my binge and I know I will have a 3 or 4 lb gain to show for it tomorrow, but thankfully I do not feel too down about it and I will have a good week next week, despite 2 meals out!!! I know I have not had a good few weeks, not been following the SW plan so much, but I will get back to it, I will do better and get the last of this weight off. I've just been well....a bit lazy about it lately.

Slimming World Week 58

Slimming World Weigh-In
Weight = 9 st 1 lb (127 lbs)
Loss = 1 lb
Lost So Far = 39 lbs
YES I LOST !!!!!!

Let's get Christmassy!!

Monday 9th December 2002

It's the Slimming World (our groups) Christmas Party tonight. And....and even though I know I will have a gain...I will still enjoy myself. (This written in advance Saturday Night)!!

Woa... I lost a lb, I really lost a pound, after all I said! I felt as light as a feather as I walked home after the meeting (funny how not many hours before I felt as fat as....HUGE cos I thought I'd gained quite a few. Bodies are SOOOOOOOOOOO weird.

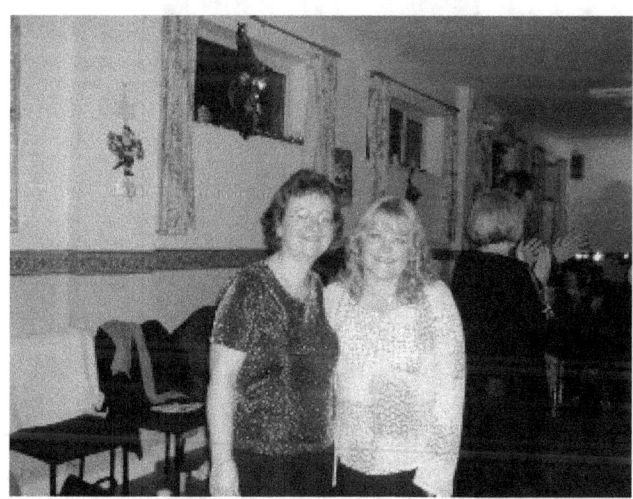

Here's me and Melanie at the Slimming World Xmas Party, everyone had a great time, the food was wonderful and we all danced loads! Mel and I are the same height and weigh the same at the moment. We have ever so slightly different Target Weights that we are aiming for....but we are both ALMOST there!

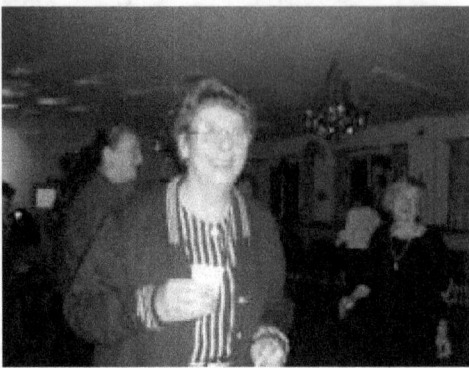

And here's Carol our Slimming World Consultant, she is so lovely and we all enjoy the meetings and walk away feeling like we CAN lose this weight and it's not so hard as you think it is!!!! I really enjoy Monday mornings doing the weigh-in with Carol.

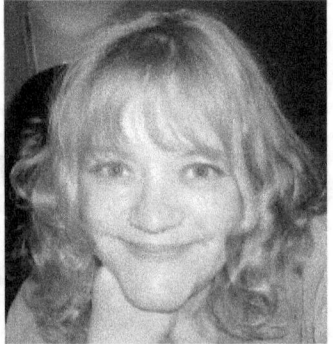

Me after the SW party. I had a great night. Our morning classes and the evening class joined up for this Party. We has loads of delicious food and everyone danced. The girl who did the disco is a singer and she also sang some songs for us, so we had a disco and live entertainment. Carol said she forgives us if we get there NEXT Monday and have had a gain - though we do have the rest of the week to be good!!!!!!!

Wednesday 11th December 2002

Went to the hospital to keep my mum company yesterday, dad was having his bypass. My sister said (today) he was off the ventilator and would come out of ICU later today. I am so glad it all went ok.

I have caught a few episodes of Ed on our channel E4 and now I am totally hooked. I think this Canadian show has been around since 2000 and is now a hit. It stars the gorgeous Tom Cavanagh . The cast of characters is likeable and I want to watch it every day! It is on 2pm ish every week day and when I am out it's a scramble for the tape to record on!!!! Tonight I am off out to my Diabetic committee Christmas meal, 3 courses! I have not eaten much so far today, just a bacon sandwich. I am looking forward to the meal (just wish it wasn't soooooooo COLD out!

Thursday 12th December 2002

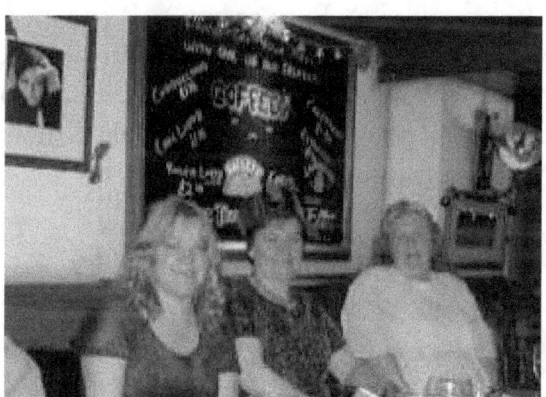

Here I am at last nights meal. It was a nice meal, there was 10 of us there altogether. I had my long red velvet dress on, mainly cos it lets me breathe out easily and is v. christmassy!!!!!!! Went out and did a bit of Xmas shopping today, did have a nibble...ok had a Twix!! Why is shopping so stressful even when you are on your own??

Slimming World Week 59

Slimming World Weigh-In
Weight This Week = 9 st 2 lbs (128 lbs)
Gain = 1 lb
Total Lost So Far = 38 lbs

Monday 16th December 2002

Got weighed today and was pleased to have only gained 1 lb. I am going to count the 'sins' properly this week, I do not want another gain right before Christmas. A one pound gain is ok this week since last week I didn't exactly follow the SW plan, what with various meals out and unplanned food here and there.

Tuesday 17th Dec 2002

Neil is off for the day, we went to Sainsbury's for breakfast (after running R to school). I had my 'red' day breakfast, v. good, then went and had some after eight mints (5 altogether....whooops, how many sins is this??) I simply must count them. Just looked them up online they are 2 sins each, so I have had 10 sins today.

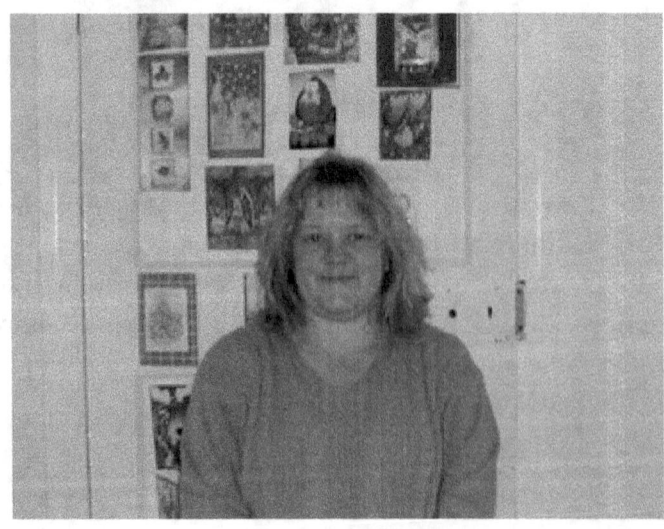

Here I am last Christmas, trying not to feel fat...wearing big baggy things and hating being the size I was...I think I was about 11 st 3 lbs (157 lbs) here

Wednesday 18th Dec 2002

Am off to the hospital today to an occupational therapy app. For an assessment on my hands. I rather overdid the sins yesterday so do not have many left for the week. If I want to have a weightloss next Monday then I will certainly have to eat better for the rest of the week. That silly picking is sneaking back in, perhaps a bit forgivable for this time of year....it is soooooooooooo easy to do!

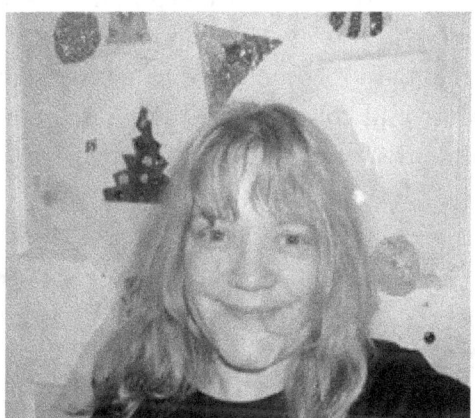

Me this Christmas feeling so much slimmer....wearing tighter clothes (better ones) and not feeling half as bad about the size I am...which is 9 st 2 lbs (128 lbs)

Happy Christmas

Slimming World Weigh-In
Weight this week = 9 st 3 lbs 129 lbs)
Gain = 1 lb (Oh it is Christmas!)
10 lbs to go to get to target

Monday 23rd December 2002

Got weighed today and have gained another lb. I do not mind too much, I know that once Xmas is over I will get back to it and it should not take me too long to get to my target weight. Mel came round for a coffee, she has done so well with losing weight and even lost another lb this week...well done! Not very many people came to get weighed this week, but I expect lots will come after Christmas! I am going to try my best to eat better (!). At least I don't drink now, that would make it even harder!

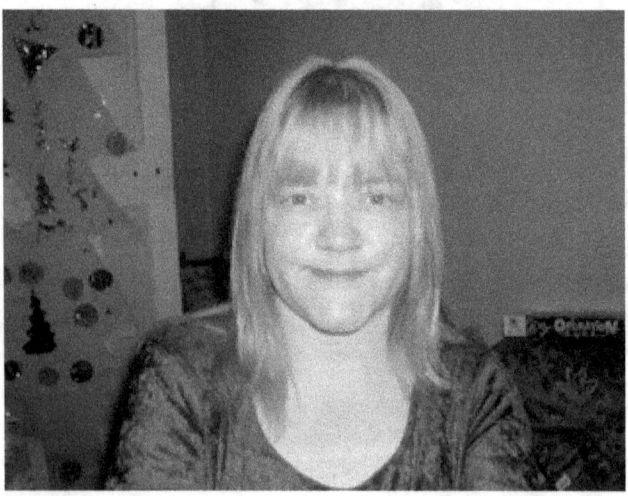

Christmas Eve

Ooooohhhhh I can feel my waist expanding as I breathe!!! Went shopping to Asda (it was mad....all elbows and shoving for sprouts at 10p a bag!!!) I got myself some bedtime jama pants for £3.50 for 2 pairs in the sale...age 15-15 and they fit!!!!!

Hopefully we will get the kids off to sleep relatively early and snuggle up to the telly and ok EAT!!! And then wrap those pressies (I am so crap at wrapping things, they always look like they have been sat on after I have spent ages trying to wrap them neatly!) Then to go to bed.

Friday 27th December 2002

Worked at the shop today. Then J met me for lunch and I was persuaded to have a ham baguette. Had made turkey and onion and carrot soup (yummy leftovers) to have at home to be good. Now Neil has come home and fancies a Chinese takeaway (which I have nicely ordered! and am waiting to be delivered as I type). God my stomach is huge.....just how many lbs have I gained???? Still... not to worry they will be gotten off!!!! I feel soooooooooooooooo stuffed now after eating all that Chinese! Tomorrow I will ease myself back into the SW diet really I will. I need to get back to eating properly, I am sure my blood sugars have been sky high for weeks now.

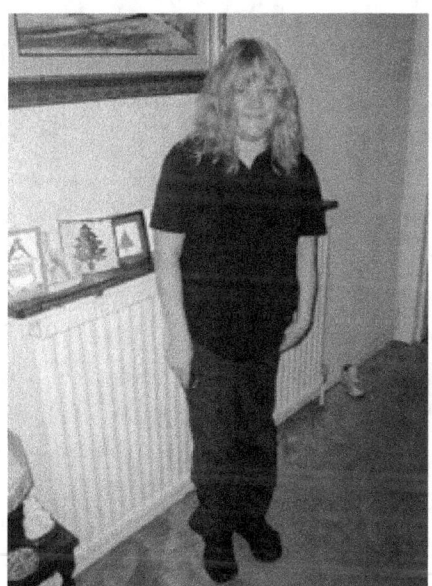

Here I am at my mother-in-laws last night

Saturday 28th December 2002

Ohhhh what good intentions... but not today. We went shopping (the start of all overeating). I bought some cream cakes and merrily (yuckily?) ate 4 of them, Neil threatened to take a pic of me eating them for the site... what a sight I was! I sat on the couch in the evening hiding under a fleecy blanket, letting it casually but intentionally cover me to hide my now looking VAST stomach (where on earth did it come from? Ah could be those creams cakes and all the stuff I ate before and during Christmas) The Slimming World Plan has gone out the window. I am desperately trying to get myself back into STICKING to the plan. So....tomorrow, I will have a RED day and aim to have well under 10 sins. I shall even get my little tub of pennies out (with my 70 sins for the week). I feel fat and sluggish and blubbery and yuck and like my body is in dire need of sorting out. And all this minus alcohol...all my 'fatness' has come about without the aid of alcohol, I cannot drink. Ok so I had some Baileys one night (3 small glasses). Heaven knows how much more weight I would have gained had I been able to drink! Neil kindly said (tonight)I was looking chubby (or words to that effect), I soooooooo wanted to crawl under the fleece and stay there to emerge some weeks later THIN...but no matter how much I try to hide my weight gain it is still there and the only thing to do is move on, tackle it and get rid of it. It may not be as much a gain as I feel....last weigh in I was 9 st 3 lbs (129 lbs), my scales say I now weigh 9 st 3 lbs these weigh 2 lb less than SW so on SW I should weigh 9 st 5 lbs - a 2 lb gain. But, I shall find out on Monday morning just how much I have gained this week. The thing being now is I need to get back on the plan and get losing this weight....I know I can do it.

Sunday 29th December 2002

Have been quite good today. Neil went out to the shop and bought cakes and some sweets, despite getting weighed in the morning and weighing in at 19 st 4 lbs (OOhhhhhhhh), that's 270 lbs. I still weigh 9 st 3 lbs on mine (129 lbs). I ate a few sweets and COUNTED them! I am pleased I managed to stick to the plan today (so far! - it's now 7.40 pm). I have my supply of Muller Light yoghurts in the fridge. Neil has just pointed out that he is just over 10 st heavier than me (oh my GOD), that's 141 lbs heavier! Oh we Sooooooooooooooo have to do something about this (and I don't mean me putting on weight!) He weighs almost the same as when he first started dieting back in March 2002, then he was 19 st 9 lbs (275 lbs)and he is now 19 st 4 lbs (270 lbs).

Slimming World Week ?

Slimming World Weigh-In
Weight This Week= 9 st 7 lbs (133 lbs)
Gain= 4 lbs
Total Lost So Far= 33 lbs (2 st 5 lbs)
Lbs to lose to target= 1 st (14 lbs)

Monday 30th December 2002

I know, I know I have gained this week...this is my last gain for now!! I am back on track and ready to get rid of the last of this weight....it HAS to go. I do not want it anymore!!

I gained 4 lbs. I didn't think it would be quite so much, but it was. I will forget about it now and move on. Yesterday I stuck to the plan and much the same today, so it's a good start.....I am aiming to lose for next week.

Tuesday 31st December 2002

Why is it that any gains go straight to your stomach and face?? Why do I always look like a moron in my photos?? Am off to sister-in-laws later hopefully she will have NO goodies on display for picking at. Kids are hoping for chocolate from her house cos we have none here! I have gone back to wondering when is the next meal and what can I eat for it (arggghhhhhhhh....hopefully as the week goes on this will fade away). I have set myself a challenge to lose 6 lbs this month (more would be better...), I want to lose that 6 lbs I gained over the Christmas periodish (over 3 weeks of not so controlled eating). Forget Christmas, it's gone, it's left me with some extra weight I do not want but...but there's the New Year Resolutions!!

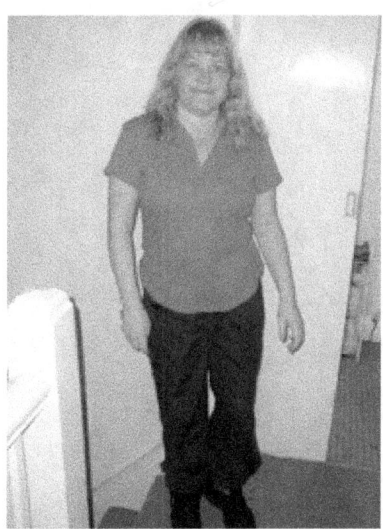

Here I am with that little old 4 lbs Christmas week gain

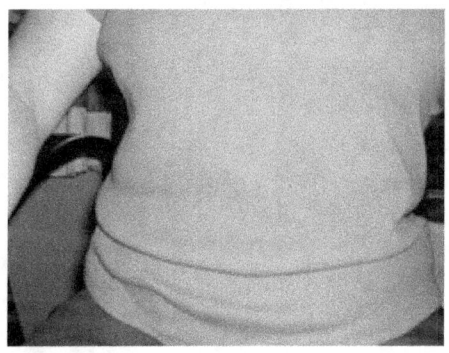

Here's that 4 lbs in close-up (hehe)! Ok I admit it, I am holding it in some! But you've got to haven't you. That's what it's all about, holding it in, makes your muscles stronger. Can't let it all hang out, slack. Get those muscles toned (somehow!). Sit ups, that's what I'll do, say 100 of them every day (to begin with), maybe not right now, I have just had breakfast!

2003

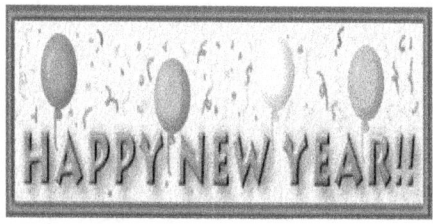

Wednesday 1st January 2003

Happy New Year everyone. Managed to stay up till about 1am watching nothing in particular on TV with Neil and J. Heard all the fireworks going off. Didn't do much today. Oh overdid the chocolates AGAIN later on and now at almost 2pm in the morning (as in Thursday 2nd) I feel sick....serves me right

Thursday 2nd January 2003

Here I am it's 2 in the morning (just beginning today), I am about to go to sleep and as I just said (see above) I feel yucky cos I grossed out on chocolate earlier while watching CSI. I was not even hungry. Now in order to have any chance of weightloss this coming Monday, I have to be soooo good with my eating from today....zero sins and free foods and the healthy A's and B's. Here goes!!!!

Friday 3rd January 2003

Can you believe I woke up (late), that's not it....well, I got downstairs and there on the kitchen table was a tub of sweets. Now last night I said to myself, NO MORE...so here I was (not even had breakfast) and I ate 2 sweets. Ok it's not a major thing, but what a waste of slimming world sins. I am going to be good. I got a letter from the hospital for my usual diabetic check-up and I have to have my hba1c (overall blood sugars level) checked and I know it will be high, and I need to get it lower, much lower...so, No more sweets! I need an exercise plan, one to do at home, an easy peasey one that I can do here and there. Will have to have a search online for such a thing.

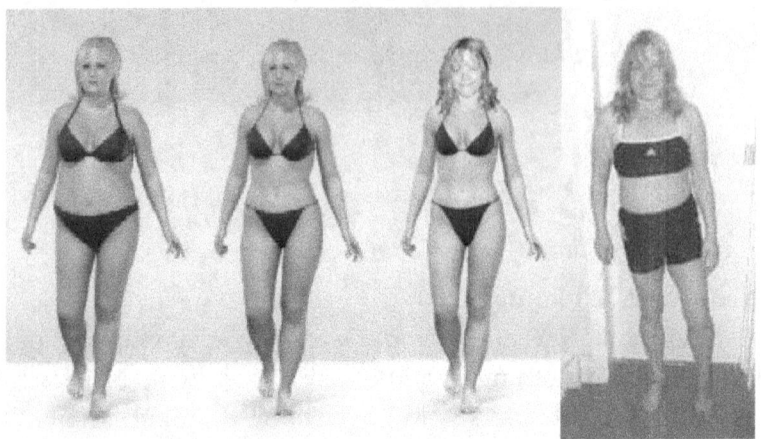

1. This is me at 133 lbs (9 st 7 lbs) (the fat is concentrated more on my stomach in real life!).
2. I want to be here at 116 lbs (8 st 4 lbs). Oh and...
3. How did this happen, here I AM at 116 lbs... gosh, I look great but perhaps in need of a tan?! OH DEAR and...
4. Here I am in real life at 127 lbs (pre Christmas grub n goodies) (I need a waist - lots of toning and a loss of 10 lbs+ oh and a sexy bikini!)

This was done with a bit of help from Neil.....he fixed my body!!

I look good don't I? Gosh even at 8 st (112 lbs) many many years ago my body never looked like this....but. perhaps with a LOT of work and exercise (hit the gym) I can at least try for it...what do you think??

Friday 3rd January Again

I won and bought (On EBay) an absolutely beautiful dress. It is so gorgeous and a size 12. Now with it coming from the US I thought it was a US 12 but it seems to be a UK 12. I am a 14... but... but I am going to lose this weight and this dress is going to fit me. At the moment I can zip it up a tiny bit of the way!. Now every time I go to the kitchen to eat something I shouldn't I am going to remember the dress. Pity

I can't hang it in the kitchen really! But on the other hand I can put a pic up of it... yes I will do that. I have so got to lose this weight and also I keep looking at my virtual model a la Cathy and I want that body...or as near enough to it as I can get. Why not. Why not go for it... aim for it... make an effort for it. I have my membership to the gym, do I use it...no not often. SO why not do myself a favour and get along there a few times a week. I am sure it will speed things up, I know it will.

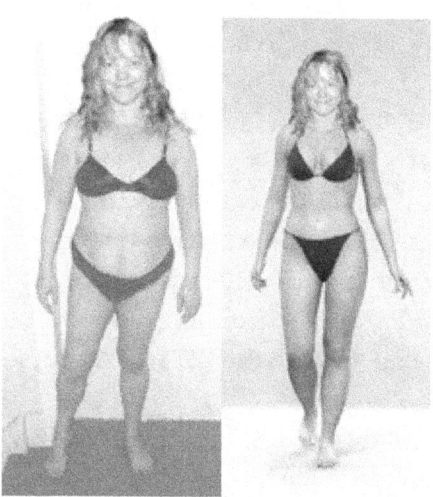

Yep here we are again with some photo manipulation. Now.....Body 1 and head 1 are totally mine (though the head is off a different photo of me, as is the body), body 2 is what I am aiming for, head 2 is mine....get it so far???? Neil says head on body 1 is a fraction too large....I say no the body is too large (hehe)...difference of opinion here!!!! Body 1 needs a better bikini top/bottom....body 2's is fine...no complaints here. So as I said pic one is all of me, though taken on different days (body was taken today, head was taken some weeks ago....but then you don't put weight on your head do you! Have no excuses for the body as such). Ah well Cathy...keep working at it!!! Enough photo trickery......now I get serious and go for it...a better body!!

Slimming World Week 62

Monday 6th January 2002

Slimming World Weigh-In
Weight = 9 st 2 lbs (128 lbs)
Loss = 5 lbs
Total Loss so Far = 38 lbs
Lbs to target = 9 lbs

Now how will I do today?? I am hoping for even a small weightloss...but I was not so good last week. Kim is joining the gym, so that makes me want to go back too. The gym do a 12 week Weightloss Course... with one to one help and an exercise programme and you have a food diary too. I think even though I am doing Slimming World I will go along on Tuesday and sign up for the 12 week course (it has got to help!)

Can you believe it I lost 5 lbs!!!! 5 lbs!!! Wow... I feel slimmer today I do!!! I AM going to have a good week and stick to the plan and if I do it properly I will be in the 8 st's by next week... have not been there for 12 years!!!

Still Monday 6th January and it is now 3.30pm. I have been thinking. One of the reasons I lose the weight is A. I do stick to the SW Plan (mainly) and by doing this I eat better. The Slimming World Plan has what are called Red Days and Green Days. On Red days you eat mainly meat - the meat (all meat) is free) and on Green Days you eat mainly pasta/rice/potatoes. Of course it is not quite as simple as this. You have lists of healthy A and B choices to have on both plans, you have to eat 1 healthy A a day and 2 healthy B's. Then you have lists of what are FREE foods on both plans and yes you can eat green day stuff on red days and vice versa (you count them as sins or healthy B's). Then of course you are allowed up to 10 sins a day, or treats you might call them. But they can be whatever you fancy. I no longer eat white bread, the whole family now eat only wholemeal bread. I rely a lot on FREE foods to fill me up and try to limit my sins. Some people save their sins for the weekend, or spread them throughout the week. It sounds complicated but it isn't. It's about eating healthier. I don't find myself thinking I am on a diet. Ok, so after Christmas (where I must admit I didn't think too closely about what I was eating)...going back to the SW Plan has not been easy peasey. But...now that I have had some days eating properly, I am finding I am enjoying my food more and eating better and I am NOT hungry. To follow any healthy eating plan you need to have the information to hand and I find going to the Slimming World meetings once a week certainly helps me (even more so because I have to go because I do the weighing, which I really enjoy). I have some of the books and I get the magazine (I love reading the success stories). So, if you are thinking about joining a slimming group/club then give it a go...what have you got to lose except weight (ok so money...if you get nowhere....but hey you'll never know till you try) And I think that if one group does not work for you try a different one.

Thursday 9th January 2003

Last 3 days I have been back to the gym. I have really enjoyed it. I have been going after I drop R at school and staying about 2 hours. My gym does a 12 week weightloss course, I have just signed up for it today. I have my first assessment next week. They will design an exercise programme for me and I have to keep a food diary (and exercise). I know I am doing Slimming World, so I will still be following this plan but I need some exercise. You get one to one advice and regular assessments and re-doing of your programme.....I am really looking forward to doing it. I did an hour in the gym the other day and then went to one of their yoga classes. I have never done yoga before and I must admit

I really enjoyed it. So I will be doing the yoga class every Wednesday. Diet wise I have been eating well, though am rather bloated cos of time of the month and overdoing the veggies!!!!! I have eaten a few things I never meant to so I think I have had too many sins but hopefully the exercise will help this????

Saturday 11th January 2003

Have been eating lots of veggies and onions! I just love onions really I do, I could eat them every day, generally I have them dry fried with other stuff with pasta. Have put a bid in on EBay for a black 1950's halter neck bikini...I hope I have won it, it is a size 12 (8 USA). That will be nice for the summer hols! I am not so bloated as I was and feel considerably thinner! I was going to go to the gym today but felt narky so did not go, probably would have felt better if I had gone. I am aiming to go for 2 hours tomorrow morning while Neil looks after the kids then I have the kids afternoon so he can do his stuff (which unfortunately is work).

Sunday 12th Jan 2003

Am not going to the gym, am going to my mums instead (Neil can get more done/peace that way). Neil has done so well the last few weeks, he lost 5 lbs last week and 4 lbs this week....this is great! Now all we have to do is keep him motivated and not bored with 'dieting'. I need to do more preparation with food, sometimes when I have nothing planned to eat it is so easy to just eat anything (which usually ends up being too fattening). I shall make more of the Slimming World recipes, I did make a few last week and have taken a liking to this Corned Beef Spaghetti Bol, it is delicious, Neil loves it too

Slimming World Week 63

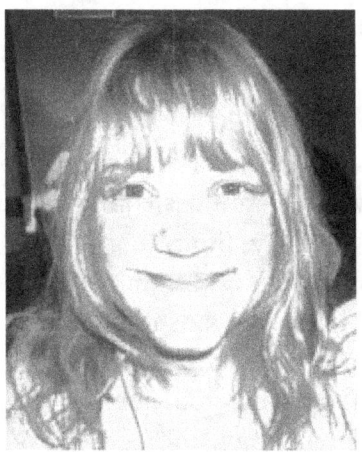

Hi Everyone.....here I am , another week. I did not eat as well as I would have wanted last week... but cannot turn back the clock now, must just try to eat healthier this week. I am not slipping back into old eating habits but it is easy to go over those sins and then find Oooppppps I have not lost weight this week. I know I can do it and I am not going to stop now, I have had many years of crappy eating and after just over a year at Slimming World my eating habits have definitely changed for the better.....some come on Cathy, get to that target!!!!!!!!!!

Monday 13th Jan 2002

Get weighed again today...I had over my sins last week but am hoping with the excrcise (went to the gym 4 times) I have stayed the same (Here's hoping!!)

Arggggggg I gained 3 lbs. I kind of knew I had, my stomach feels so bloated. I overdid the 'sins' last week, despite doing 3 days of the gym and it's almost period time and well.....never mind. Thing is, nowadays I do not get down about gains, I just move on. I am now going to have a GOOD week and stick to the plan. (That's the plan!!!!)

Slimming World Weigh-In
Weight = 9 st 5 lbs (131 lbs)
Gain = 3 lbs
Total Lost so Far = 2 st 7 lbs (35 lbs)
Lbs to go to Target = 12 lbs

Wednesday 15th January 2003

Had a fitness assessment at the gym today (have signed up for their 12 week weightloss course). I am UNFIT, really I am, though am slightly fitter than I was when I had an assessment at my heaviest weight! It will improve (I hope). My BMI is 25.7, I know it needs to be under 24. I am planning on going to the gym Tues/Weds/Thurs and one of the weekend days. They said you need to go a minimum of 3 times a week. I also have a food diary to fill in. I am determined this time to get going again and get rid of the last of this weight, I feel that by going back to the gym this will most certainly help this along. I have been going to yoga and have been to tone and stretch classes, both are really good and I enjoy them. I have been a member of the gym for just over 2 years now and have hardly been there at all the last 12 months, now I need to get my money's worth!!

Friday 17th Jan 2003

Wouldn't you know it...I won a huge tin of sweets at the local hospital tombola...and am desperate for them to be all eaten and gone. Oh I have had my fair share of them....far too many and I doubt very much if all my gym visits will cancel them out (yet again). How stupid can you be. I have put a load in a bag for my mother and father in law (the sweets we are not keen on, but can eat if that was all there was left... so they can go at least!) I am taking J to see Die Another Day (007) at the cinema tomorrow so he can have some for munchies there...unless Neil finishes them off tonight?! I am planning on going to the gym for an hour in the morning and on Sunday morning, I would not be going this much except I ate all these chocolates (silly me).

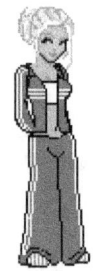

How I would like to look at the gym, but don't!

Saturday 18th January 2003

Went to the cinema and ate ok a few sweets...not too many mind. Though it was lunchtime so I had a children's McDonalds (wanted the toy!) Was good otherwise.

Sunday 19th January 2003

Neil has gained weight this week, but then I did go and win those chocolates so he is forgiven! This coming week I am going to cook cook cook and we are both going to get this weight off. Neil does need all the help he can get. Though he is very good when he is at work (at the office), it's when he gets home that 'stress' kicks in/temptation is there/boredom/free access to the kitchen/late night eating when I am in bed (Neil not me! I sleep ...can't eat when you are asleep) Neil has this awful habit of rarely sleeping... or avoiding it as long as he can... no wonder is he knackered at work. The downside of this is he goes to the kitchen and snacks.

Slimming World Week 64

Slimming World Weigh-In
Weight = 9 st 4 lbs (130 lbs)
Loss = 1 lb
Total Lost So Far = 2 st 8 lbs (36 lbs)
Lbs Left to Target = 11 lbs

Monday 20th January 2003

Well as you can see I have lost a lb, which is good. Watched a programme on women and men who had lost a lot of weight (with slimming clubs) only to gain it all back and usually more. No way hose-a am I going to gain my weight back. I am getting used to the slimmer me now and actually am feeling fatter now so the new me needs to lose that last lot of weight, if you see what I mean?! My stomach certainly does not wobble half as much and things stay in place more and I like it!!!

Friday 24th January 2003

I have been eating chocolate again (why why why why????????). So here's a bloody awful photo of me to remind me of why I should not be eating SOOOOOOOOOOOOO much chocolate. Eat some yes......but quite so much NO.

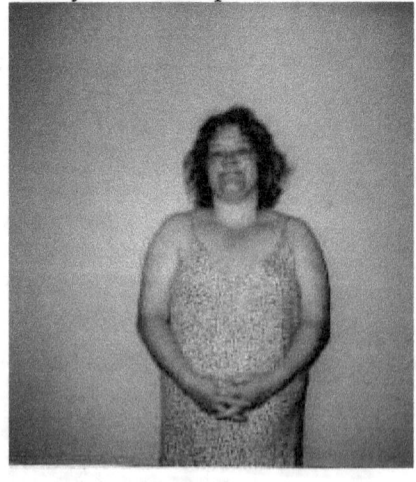

I am doing all the right things otherwise. I am following the SW Plan (apart from the extras!), I have been going to the gym 3 + times a week and making my self work harder when I am there). So why do I spoil it?? Now I feel bloated and sick and fat and tired. I am going to the gym tomorrow and Sunday and I will work that bit harder to make up for all the chocolate I ate today. Yet again I know I will not lose weight his coming week...I disappoint myself. But...but, I am still determined to do it properly and I am feeling positive despite the setbacks (despite my lack of willpower). I am doing the 12 week weightloss course at the gym and I am going to have a good 12 weeks and be fitter/slimmer at the end of it (and hopefully more toned!!). We all have bad weeks, sometimes these weeks go on longer than I'd really like but I WILL do BETTER.

Sunday 26th January 2003

Well here I am on Sunday night at 10.44 pm. Yesterday we went out to see the Historic Warships (The Plymouth which went to the Falklands and a sub, can't remember what it was called....very Voyage To The Bottom Of The Sea). We rushed out (was getting late in the day) I grabbed a load of rather unhealthy snacky things from Tesco (as you do...for the kids). And I managed to eat a donut/a kit-kat and some mini eggs, chocolate ones of course. (Well done Cathy). It was a nice afternoon out...though I wish I hadn't eaten all those things. So here I am feeling the worse for eating , funny how they can tell on your stomach so quickly?? I won't despair no matter how much I have gained tomorrow ('sfunny, I have been saying this a lot lately) OK so it's not funny at all really. I feel....I am feeling curvy (too curvy!!!)

Slimming World Week 65

Monday 27th January 2003

I am not really looking forward to getting weighed today. I have eaten so badly this last week. I will...I will have a better week this week. What is the point of me going to the gym and Slimming World if I don't make an effort with the eating?? But, we all have bad weeks don't we and the point is not to give up. As you can see I gained 2 lbs. This has to stop... here... now. I cannot, simply cannot gain anymore weight...I will not gain anymore weight. I have started today off well (apart from that gain!) and I am going to have a GOOD week. SO THERE!!

Slimming World Weigh-In
Weight = 9 st 6 lbs (132 lbs)
Gain = 2 lbs
Total Lost so Far = 34 lbs

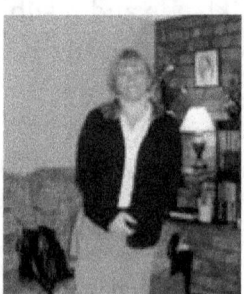

Here I am today, after the weigh-in

I am a jelly. I feel like a jelly, I look like a jelly...therefore I am a jelly (at least round my middle). It is not fair!

The stretch class is so good, I really feel it, and there is no bounding around but you work very hard. My body needs all the toning and stretching it can get.

Tuesday 28th January 2003

Well I ate ok yesterday. Neil pointed out that I made a spelling mistake on yesterdays bit...saying I was going to have a good wee! I meant week of course, but I do have a good wee before I get weighed, don't think it makes a difference really but it makes me feel it does!! Today I did some work in the gym and then went to the tone and stretch class which I really enjoyed.

Thursday 30th Jan 2003

I have been working quite hard at the gym and have also been going to a lot of the various classes, which I am enjoying. I have eaten much better this week....though the biscuits are beckoning at the moment (Neil bought some yummy ones for the kids tonight on the way home) But... I will do my best to resist. If I have not lost weight when I go on Monday I will be most cross.

Friday 31st Jan 2003

I was going to have a Chinese tonight, spoke to Neil on AIM and he wants some...but now I have lost my appetite (which is just as well perhaps). I have only got 6 sins left for the whole weekend. I am aiming to go to the gym on Sunday. I have been saying this for the last few weeks (that I will go at the weekend) but somehow have never got there. But this weekend I will go if it is ok with Neil. I think I need to work harder at the gym and thankfully my joints are holding up pretty good, though I have been waking up in the middle of the morning with my hands really hurting which is fixed with a few painkillers. I need to push myself more... to do more at the gym. Just feel a bit down at the moment.

Had the Chinese in the end, was as good with it as I could be! I hope. Now I have to be terribly good for the rest of the weekend. And yes I can do that bit extra at the gym on Sunday morning for any overdoing it!

Saturday 1 February 2003

Well took the kids out for the day so Neil could do some work. Wanted to buy myself some chocolate (but didn't) and had 2 sticks of liquorice instead which is not as bad. I do not know if I have lost weight this week...I must say I feel as if I have, but I have been eating too many snacky things and biscuits...I really must limit this as much as possible.

Am still wanting a 1940's makeover for my 40th birthday this year. I have the Grace Kelly dress (ok it doesn't fit yet but it will), by then I will probably have something different to wear!! But I want (the....a...any) gorgeous dress (1940's style) and the hair do and make-up to go with it...and ok the photo at the end of it to show off my weightloss (which when i get to goal will be almost 4 stone or round about 50 lbs)

Sunday 2nd February 2003

Neil has lost 2 lbs this week. We have to go for it and make more of an effort too...so that Neil can finally lose this weight. I do not know how I have done this week... well, I do a bit, I have eaten too many sins and gone over the plan, so in reality I should not have lost weight, on the other hand I have been doing a lot of exercise so this may have helped (I hope it has helped) I went to the gym today (Kim rang and I went with her). The in the afternoon I helped the kids do chocolate, I had bought some moulds and we melted the choccy and so on. Good job the chocolate was not that nice or I would have eaten more!!

Slimming World Week 66

I am feeling watery!

Monday 3rd Feb 2003

I wonder how the weigh-in will go today? I just do not know.

Slimming World Weigh-In
Weight = 9 st 2 lbs (128 lbs)
Loss = 4 lbs
Total Lost So Far = 38 lbs
Lbs to go to target = 9 lbs left to go

Yes...yes...yes....I lost 4 lbs, I am so pleased. I am desperate almost to get under 9 st, only I can do it....I know I can do it. I am sticking to this healthy eating plan and I am not hungry, the only thing that lets me down is the bad snacking (over and above what is allowed in order to lose weight each week).

Yes I CAN do it

Tuesday 4th February 2003

Have 2 classes today, aerobics and tone and stretch. The aerobics was very hard, they used the step and I am not so good on this (found it hard to keep up) plus it knackers my knees a bit.....so I might avoid this class till I am fitter.

Wednesday 5th February 2003

Today I did my tone and stretch class (yes again) and the yoga class. Got weighed at the gym and was heavier than at SW....but well...different scales and all that, but it certainly does not help your motivation. Had a medical at my GP's (so I can apply for my provisional driving licence) arghhhhhhhhh he said "You have cataracts yes" I said NO....but he said yes I did and had I not been told? NO I HADN'T. What? Where (I know where)? How? Why? I thought only old people got them (god this is not going to be a good year what with my 40th birthday!! Still....I AM going to get to my target weight, I AM going to get a job, I AM (probably/hopefully) going to pass my driving test!! Oh ok I went and had some chocolate tea-cakes at my mother-in-laws after the medical cos I felt sorry for myself and later on tonight I had a packet of crisps (but) but that is all.......mini self pity binge over with! There are worse ailments to have and I am getting fitter really I am.....al this gym work has got to be doing me good. Apart from being a bit tired now and then in the afternoons, generally my energy has gone up, I, overall am less tired (I think), though Neil will thoroughly disagree with this when I say I am off to bed (and it's only 9pm!!!!).

Friday 7th Feb 2003

Ohhh I feel fat and bloated and flabby and it's not fair. This is definitely going to be one step forward and 2 back weight wise. I seem to have a good week then a not so good week. I have the desperation to do it (lose the last of this weight) but not the 'get up and go' at the moment. Well...at least I am keeping up with the gym and working quite hard at it. We are off to (of all places) Cadburys Chocolate Factory (Cadburyland) tomorrow! Now...how good can I be? I am taking my own lunch (Neil said "oh you've gotta eat out on a day out". We shall see...I am to do the least damage as possible. I know the kids (and Neil probably) will get yummily sick on chocolate!) I have visions of Willy Wonkas Chocolate Factory......it's in a place called Bourneville too!!!

Sunday 9th Feb 2003

I never want to see another piece of chocolate ever again! We got to Cadbury World an hour late, by which time I was mega stressed, R was crying and J was moaning. Rang my friend who finally directed us to the right place (had been trying to phone the Cad World but it was constantly engaged). Kim said...go eat some chocolate! So I did....they gave everyone loads, everywhere you turned they gave you chocolate!!!! Ate in their cafe and had a salad!!!! So....combined with a not so good rest of the week...how much will I have gained tomorrow (and that's not even with the chocolate catching up with me).

Slimming World Week 67

Monday 10th February 2003

I know, I just know I have gained weight this week and I am so fed up with myself. I know what to do to get back on track and I must make an effort and do it. I don't want to get to the Summer Hols and find I am the same weight as now. I felt so fat yesterday (especially after all that chocolate). And I keep seeing myself in the mirrors at the gym and cringing (just how many spare tyres do I have? Too many). So........I have to change this.

Slimming World Weigh-In
Weight = 9 st 4 lbs (130 lbs)
Gain = 2 lbs
Total Lost So Far = ermm...2 st 8 lbs 9 that's 36 lbs)

Tuesday 11th February 2003

I knew I had....anyway I gained 2 lbs. I am good at this 2 on 2 off business!! I simply must get below 9 st (126 lbs). I (reluctantly) looked at myself in the gym mirrors today (arhhhghghghg) and I must admit my shape is far better (is improving)....things don't look half as flabby. So whilst I am not doing great things weightloss wise, I must be doing some good going to the gym 3 and 4 times a week. I do a tone and stretch class on a Tuesday morning followed by about half an hour in the gym (more if I am feeling up to it!), then I do a tone and stretch class on a Wednesday morning followed by a yoga class, then on Thursdays I do a arobatone class followed by some gym work....then if I am not too tired (and Neil is ok...as in not working) I go and do an hour to 2 hours in the gym on a Sunday too. PHEW!!!! I have been doing this for the past 3 to 4 weeks.

Thursday 13th February 2003

Am feeling Soooooooooooooooo FAT...totally totally FAT and flabby and fed up. I did not go to the gym today, I felt so yuck and not in the mood, so I more or less slept from 10am to 2pm...took to my bed as it were. I then made an effort and went out, just to the shops, but I went out. I hate days (times like this). I am planning on going to the gym at the weekend, perhaps this will make me feel better. Tomorrow I work in the shop (I work 9am-1pm on Fridays in Oxfam on the till), I quite enjoy it. I do want a part-time job eventually, in the meantime I am trying to get some confidence workwise and get fitter at the gym.

Slimming World Week 68

Monday 17th February 2003

Well here we are again! Another week...and how do I think I have done this week??? Well, I know I have gained again, but I AM NOT GOING TO GIVE UP.

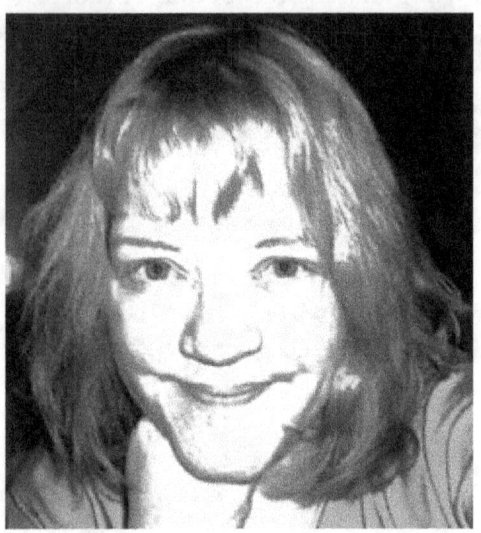

Here I am with my new haircut and a bit of playing around with Adobe Photoshop! (Covers up wrinkles!)

YES YES YES...I lost 3 lbs this week, really I did. I didn't know what to expect when I stepped on the scales and I know I have to have a good week...I want to report that I am in the 8st's next week ok!!!!!

Slimming World Weigh-In
Weight = 9 st 1 lb (127 lbs)
Loss = 3 lbs
Weight Loss So Far = 39 lbs (2 st 11)

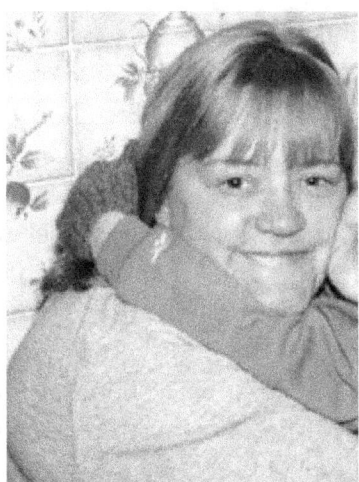

Here I am in Nov 2000, I remember wearing this big sweatshirt to cover me up.......now if I breathe in enough I can feel my ribs, see them even!!! And I have discovered my hipbones and shoulder bones!! Hips bones are the best, they are so weird to feel (not being funny here!), they stick out so, can't stop feeling them really I can't! Ok, gotta do some work on my stomach, that's still a bit too much there...but is almost flat when I am lying down!!! Before, when I lay down is was still a huge hill. I think I was very hilly back then!

Thursday 20th February 2003

Went to the gym yesterday and had my measurements done...there is 5 and a half inches less of me!! Mainly off the hips (yippee)..just gotta work on the stomach! Did my yoga class yesterday and a tone and stretch class. I think I get more out of the classes than just plodding away in the gym. Kids are off school for the week (my stress levels rise!). I am doing ok with my eating at the moment, though had a not so good start to the week...I am trying to correct this. I do find that when the kids are off school I get more inclined to head for the kitchen and eat (biscuits mainly)...I am trying not to do this (not having them in helps...the biscuits that is). I am trying not to head for the kitchen and only go in there for tea/coffee!!

Friday 21st Feb 2003

Had a break from the kids and worked at the shop. Took my Grace Kelly 'style' dress into the shop to show everyone. As I have said before, I am 40 this year (August) and I plan on having my photo done with me wearing a 40's style dress (with the hairdo and the make-up). Most people who I say this to...well I think they think I am mad?? It is just something I want to do. It may not be with the GK dress I have, I may find another dress, I do not know. And I may not lose enough weight to get into the GK dress? Though I certainly hope I do. I will have to make sure I am at target for my birthday and have been maintaining it for some time. I have (as of last Monday's weigh -in, 8 lbs to go to my target of 8 and a half stone. I may lower my target and aim to go as near to 8 st (112 lbs) as possible. Anyway first things first, let's get to 8 and a half (119 lbs).

Slimming World Week 69

Have I really been doing SW this long? YES! And I will keep going till I get to my target and afterwards...to maintain. Then hopefully by then healthier eating (and the exercise) will be more of a way of life (and less bad habits that will lead me to pile on the lbs!!

Monday 24th February 2003

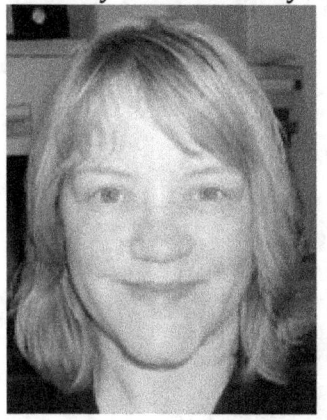

I have no idea whatsoever how I have done this week...will I make it into the 8 st's?? Did I eat properly last week or did I overdo the 'sins' on the Slimming World Plan? I bought a nice long denim skirt the other day)off a charity shop), very long, from Richards. The tag said size 12, so I figured it would fit, I can get into MOST 12's (ok not all) and anyway, I am still losing weight. So, got home and tried it on. I could only fasten 1 button, I felt so cross. Am I chubbier than I thought, are Richard shops clothes that much smaller?? I hung the skirt up and stared at it angrily. Hummph...no eating for a week! (Just kidding). How come I can only fasten 1 just 1 button??? Yesterday I bemoaned the fact to Neil....got the offending skirt out of the wardrobe and 'growled' at it. I want to get into it, it is a size 12. Tried it on again just in case (either I had altered or the skirt had??). No, yet again I could only fasten 1 button, and unfortunately it has 6 buttons to fasten down the side of the skirt). I looked at the horrid horrid label. OH MY GOODNESS....that's why, that's why it does not fit. It was a size 8. A size 8....WOW and I managed to fasten a button!!!!!!!!! Couldn't breathe of course. But I fastened a button, the top button no less!!!!!! It's a lovely skirt...and I may yet get into it, though the lowest size I have ever been is a 10.

Oh, Neil and I went out for a meal on Saturday night, I was relatively good, sort of. Only had a chicken starter, a beef sizzler main course (no rice) and ok I had a vanilla crunchie sundae for pudding...no alcohol and I had no room to finish my latte! Arrrrrrrr....forgot about that little visit to McDonalds with the kids at the beginning of the week (kids off school, half term)...well, I only had a kids meal, so not so bad. (Am writing this Sunday night...so we shall see how I do tomorrow morning eh!)

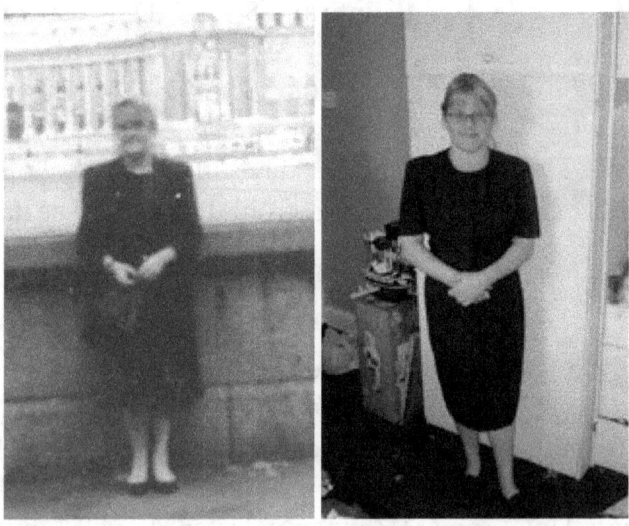

The first photo was taken in 1989 and I was in London, I had just been for an interview with Mrs Norman Tebbit (the politician's wife). She was in a wheelchair as a result of a bomb explosion in Brighton. I, at this time in 89 was registered with a Care Agency and had had a phone call to go for an interview at the Tebbits' home in London. (I didn't get the job by the way). I had bought this smart navy dress for the interview, a size 12. I thought I looked very nice! Now...all these years the dress has not even gone near me... could not even meet across my bust!!! Ah but now.....it fits, it fits again as you can see in photo 2 (the sleeves are longer in photo 1 cos I had a jacket on).

Monday 24th Feb 2003

> Slimming World Weigh-In
> Weight This Week = 9 st 2 lbs (128 lbs)
> Gain = 1 lb
> Total Lost So Far = 38 lbs
> Lbs left to lose? = about 10 lbs

Well, as you can see when I got weighed this morning I gained a lb. I was a bit disappointed, though not surprised, since I ate out this week and picked etc. I have had a good day so far (it is now 6.15pm) and I have had no sins so far today. I had fruit for brekky and sin free sausage and fruit for lunch. I want to have a good week and have a chance of getting into the 8st's next Monday. So I will do the best I can this week.

Tuesday 25th Feb 2002

Went to the gym this morning and did a tone and stretch class. Felt rather yucky later on when I got home. In fact felt sick. Father-in-law said he would get R from school for me, I wen to bed. Later discovered father-in-law had got R early from school as the secretary rang to say R had been sick. I think it is one of those 'stomach' bugs. I ate very little today (good) but munched on mints in the evening (not so good). Now I feel sick again. I may have to keep R off school tomorrow so will not be able to go to my usual classes??

Thursday 27th Feb

Had both kids off yesterday, puking and I joined in too. Today feel like someone has stomped on all my joints and churned up my stomach. Ate next to nothing yesterday, it was all I could do to sip tea.

Friday 28th Feb 2003

Worked at the shop today, had a good morning. J is still off school feeling sick. Am trying very hard not to pick (but not managing so good). It is a VERY very hard habit to get out of, really it is, especially when you have been doing it all your life! I have not been able to go to the gym this week, so I must be that extra bit careful about what I am eating (ha....is it too late?) I bought a lovely dress today (sort or 40's/50's/60's style (I do not know!!)..shall have to put it on and get piccy taken and online. I think Neil will say 'what on earth did you get that for'? or words to that effect since it is me that speaks like that not him! They are all eating a pizza/chips/burger takeaway...which is why I am up here on the computer! I did have a huge bowl of 'free' pasta beforehand so I might be full and resist. But why is it that even when you are mega stuffed you can still find room for those yummy things you ought not to eat (if you want to lose weight that is)?????? Ok I admit it I had a few chips (just a few) and I ran out of the room to avoid the smell of the garlic bread (yum)....I hastily ate a Muller yoghurt (free), even though I didn't quite want one really, but so as to avoid the chips (Mmmmmm chips dipped in yoghurt) (or fries as they are called in the US)

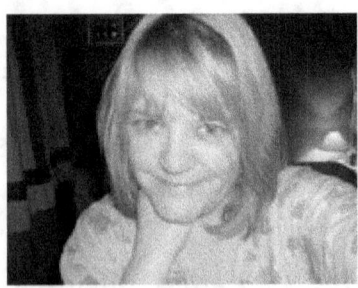

Saturday 1st March 2003

Went to my mums today, went to my sister's too, she is following SW. She has bought an air strider (wow it is great, very easy) I used up 150 calories in no time (cancelled out those few Rolos I ate at her house). I want an air walker/strider thing, bit big though, where on earth would I put it??

Gadgets are great....but you can get fed up of them, though I love my dishwasher!

Slimming World Week 70

Saturday 1st March 2003

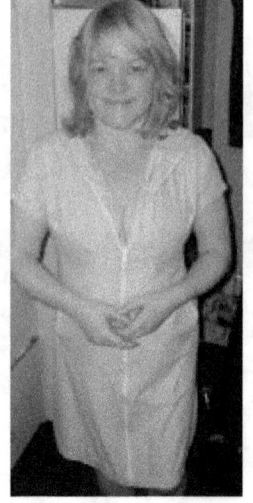

Here I am in a little tan number (ah that looks a little like a waitress uniform, but isn't!!) It's yep, a size 10 and it fits (just... but that's the style of it, no?). Looked lovely on the hanger but Mmmm, not too sure in real life (i.e. wearing it), it has a hood and pockets. Neil says I am vain (all these photos I take of myself). Ok maybe I am a little, but in truth, I take all the photos in the hope there will be one really good one...the ONE that will make me look skinny. The one photo that will make me look pretty perhaps? Tall (nah...maybe not!). I do constantly check my face for wrinkles and get quite paranoid about them. I must admit I have 3 mirrors in my hall... on the other hand, I rather like mirrors, old ones. Mirrors that look antique. Funny really when you think about how I DID avoid mirrors when I was fatter, full length ones anyway. And, and, all these photos, you do realise don't you, that for every one I put online there are 4 others that go with each one, these are the one's I deleted off the camera because I looked FAT or LUMPY, you know. gross.......so I only put the well, carefully staged (and stomach held -in) ones online.

Monday 3rd March 2003

Slimming World Weigh-In
Weight = 9 st 2 lbs 128 lbs)
Stayed the same
Total Lost So Far = 2 st 10 lbs (38 lbs)

How have I done today?? As you can see I have stayed the same, which is good, on the other hand if I stopped this picking and stuck to the plan properly... I would be losing the weight. So come on...get to it. Our Slimming World Consultant Carol is leaving on the 17th, this is sad news, she is so lovely and I have really enjoyed doing the weighing for her. We will get someone else and I expect I will continue to weigh people, which I do enjoy doing. I may consider training to be a SW Consultant myself? It all comes down to confidence. I have it...sort of!! I have lots of ideas for motivation. I can picture myself doing the job I think? I would feel happier knowing more as it were, knowing more about the plan (should go back to my books I was given when I first joined). You do get lazy and need to go back to basics sometimes.

This week I am going to:

- Stick to the plan
- Avoid picking
- Do more exercise
- Try a new SW recipe

Tuesday 4th March 2003

I know it is only Tuesday but so far I am sticking to the plan, I have eaten well and have not done any silly picking. Though I was in danger yesterday with a load of cookies!! Went to my tone and stretch class today and did an hour in the gym too. Ok, it is 20 mins to 1 in the morning and I have gotten through today without eating too much. I made some pancakes and had 3...it's ok I counted them, 2 sins each (off the Slimming World site)! I am going to the gym tomorrow, a tone and stretch class and yoga.

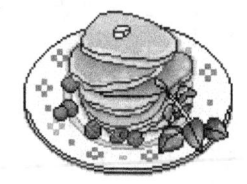

Happy Pancake Day!

Wednesday 5th March 2003

Arghhhhhhhh my feet, my feet are killing me. Today I went to the gym (lots of treadmill and yoga) and then tonight I went to my first ever Line Dancing class!!!! I must admit I really enjoyed it, it's like a challenge to get those steps right....no matter what! trouble is my body moved one way and my feet stayed where they were as I had crappy shoes on that stuck to the floor!

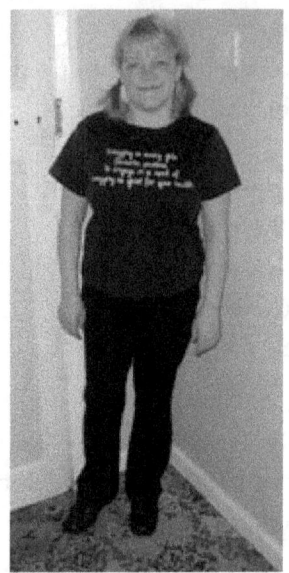

Just before my Line Dancing Class!

Thursday 6th March 2003

Exercise, exercise, exercise! My RailWalker (like and air walker/strider) came today. It's great. Unfortunately Neil is about 40 lbs+ (2 and a half stone +) too heavy to use it, but when he gets to a weight where he can use it, I will make him go on it!! It's amazing just how many calories you can burn on it. I shall be ever so fit and healthy (I hope!). Did more than usual at the gym today....then felt very tired this afternoon. Neil was off work cos he had been to physio yesterday and was hurting Soooo much (he has been diagnosed with a 'mild degenerative disease', arthritis I guess?). Now he has to have a course of physio. I wish I could help more with his weightloss, I am sure all pains will get much better when he loses weight, we simply have to get his weight down. He has not been weighed for quite a few weeks (ok, will get that battery for the scales!). For the moment we will go slowly, especially since he is in so much pain and more inclined to comfort eat.

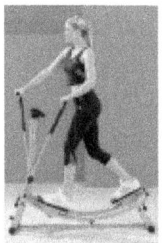

Here is the Rail Walker

Saturday 8th March 2003

Went swimming with R and friend Nicola and her daughter (J is on a camping trip with Scouts). Haven't been swimming since last Summer hols. Mind you, didn't do a lot of swimming with R in her rubber ring, but, it was fun and I really enjoyed it. Don't I sound the energetic one! Mind you I then proceeded to eat 2 Cadburys cream eggs later, and a burger + a few fries from McDonalds...so now I have to go on the railwalker tonight to undo the damage. Felt I looked soooooooo much better in my swimsuit (don't look pregnant now!!). My holderinnerupper swimsuit was a little baggy!

Sunday 9th March 2003

I am managing to resist the tin of chocolate biscuits in the kitchen, really I am. I know that if I have one of them I will end up eating LOADS. I am just about to make some lunch (am starving), a corned beef bolognaise (free) .How quickly you can go from feeling ok to not. I suddenly feel very fat and HUGE and yuck. And definitely NOT looking forward to getting weighed in the morning. I feel it's one step forward two steps back all the time. I feel a bit of a failure at the moment if I am honest. I was going to be so good this week, yet thinking back....I was not, oh I forgot about those odd biscuits here and there, those few sweets, that odd crisp here and there, that McDonalds, those 2 cream eggs, those few too many options drinks. Ah you see, when you think of all that... NO WAY can I weigh less on the scales tomorrow. No amount of exercising can undo all that. Oh well... guess I have to go get weighed, face the fact that I have done it again (or not done it!) And resolve to do better this coming week and therein.

Slimming World Week 71

Monday 10th March 2003

I wonder how I have done today (I always say this!). I stayed the same, which is good, but I need to do better. I need to have a good week, a good weightloss.

> Slimming World Weigh-In
> Weight= 9st 2 lbs (128 lbs)
> Stayed the same
> Total Lost So Far= 38 lbs
> Lbs to go to target= 9 lbs

Tuesday 11th March 2003

Well, I did my tone and stretch class today, it was ok, but felt really tired all day, almost fell asleep on the couch and overslept for getting r off school. I am aiming to go on the railwalker for 15 mins each evening, though did not do it last night cos my hands were hurting so much and making me feel yuck. Generally my arthritis is being ok (thanks to the higher dose of Methotrexate). I have being following the plan and eating ok... though it is hard to resist those chocolate biscuits in the jar. I had 2 yesterday but counted them.

Friday 14th March 2002

Today is red nose day. I did my hair red for the shop! Any excuse to dress up or do something different! I am going out tonight to the gym's 21st celebration disco with Kim. I have this red dress I really want to wear but it is sleeveless and I feel a bit lumpy in it, or rather I feel I look lumpy in it. I have another dress to choose from too, a purpley one , can't decide which to wear! I feel I look so much better but I still hate the way my stomach looks, though I know very skinny people who moan about how 'fat' their stomachs look! I have been very good despite Neil coming home last night with donuts, cherry bakewell cakes and chocolate. I was SOOOOOOOOOOOOOOO tempted, ok I admit it I had a kit-kat (a single chunky one). I ate my grapes and Muller lite yog and felt good. But when I came in today from the shop the damn donuts and cakes were there, they were there waiting to be eaten and I SO much wanted to eat them....all of them, but I didn't even have a nibble, not one teeny weeny nibble. There is a buffet tonight and I am hoping there will be 'red day' food I can eat and I am not going to have any alcohol (alcohol and me do not go together!) I can handle the odd glass or 3 but that is it. And I want to lose weight this week so am not even having 1 glass, not one.

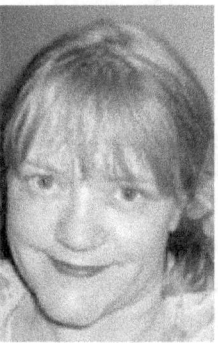

This is with my hair sprayed red
So... I went and did it reddish permanent!

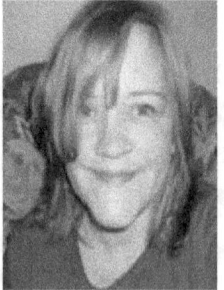

well, it is sort of reddish!

Saturday 15th March 2003

Had a good night out last night. It was packed and everyone was dancing (or standing by the bar!). There was a great buffet and I stuck to meats (red day!) and had just one lager, and the 'as you walk in' free glass of bubbly stuff. Am off to my mums today (Neil can work... poor thing!... but at least in peace). I wonder what they will say about my new hair colour? Probably won't even notice!

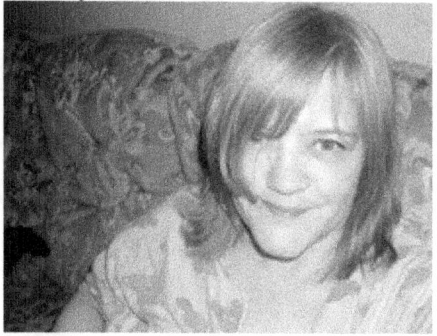

I have no idea how I might have done this week. I have resisted lots of goodies and done exercise (except Wednesday when I felt ill). Hopefully the exercise I have done will cancel out the chocolate thingies. I did have 2 choccy biscuits last night before I went out (in case of hypos and all that dancing I was going to do!). I shall have to be good in my mums and sisters. Carol our slimming world consultant is leaving on Monday, I know we will all miss her, she is so lovely.

Sunday 16th March 2003

Well, what was I saying about being good yesterday? Actually I was great in my mums and sisters, it was on the way home I was BAD. We called at the shops and I had a choccy attack and had ermmmm...some mini eggs, lots of pieces of toblerone and, oh that was it...Aghghghghghhhhhhh! I did go on the railwalker later on but barely burned up 100 calories. Today we went to a craft centre and there was a cute farm attached to it. There was this ever so cute pig, huge he was, walking around (you could 'pet' him). He was so huge (I know just how he felt!). I had a lemon ice-cream, very lemony very yummy. Then tonight I have been making nibbles for a 'taster' do at SW tomorrow. Sin free Doritos (pasta sheets boiled, cut into triangles then baked in oven) along with a low sin cheese and onion dip. So of course I tasted tonight, just to be sure. I bought some Greek yoghurt (I thought it was 0% fat...added sweetener to it, MMmmmmmmmm gorgeous with dipped fruit) but no...I got the wrong sort, the full fat one, too many sins for it, didn't I. So I gave it all to Neil to eat! Ok, I had some! Needless to say I DO feel very fat at the moment, hope this goes away by tomorrow morning.

Slimming World Week 72

Monday 17th March 2003

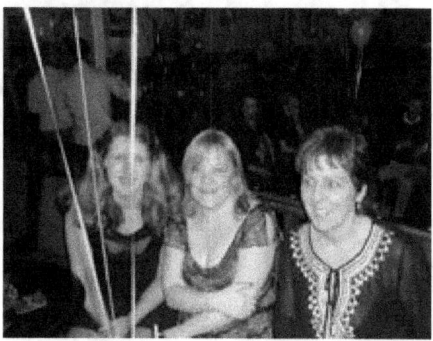

Here I am with some friends on the gym's night out. I enjoyed it and had a dance and didn't eat too much on the buffet!

YES YES YES I lost 2 lbs.....whoa and the scales flickered briefly on 8 st 13 lbs (just flickered on and off, but ummmmm stayed on 9 st exactly) But I am so pleased. We has our taster morning and it was nice, took some photos cos it was Carol's last day as our Slimming World Consultant, which was sad.

Slimming World Weigh-In
Weight = 9 st (126 lbs)
Loss = 2 lbs
Total Lost So Far = 40 lbs
Lbs to go to Target = 7 lbs

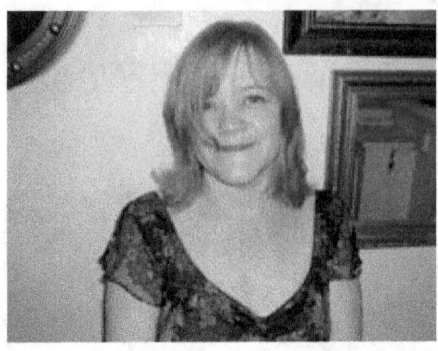

Here I am ready to go out on Friday night. I felt good in my dress, though I admit to wearing holderinnerknickers (well...I still have some weight to lose!)

Tuesday 18th March 2003

Today my mum and sister (youngest) are supposed to be visiting? So of course I am rushing round the house tidying (as you do).I say supposed to be coming, as quite often they change their minds at the last minute. Well, I got through yesterday without going over my 'sins'....so let's see how I do today. Put some new photos on the Regular photos page, not the best of photos. I was trying on dresses and unfortunately I think I need to be a foot taller!!

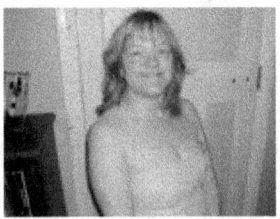

Am giving the gym a miss cos of visitors (hope they get here after all this). Housework is as good as a gym workout (well.....sort of, I do stop for coffee rather too often!)

It would be very nice to be able to look elegant in a dress. I feel I look well.......squashed!! Perhaps losing that last 10 lbs or so will take away the squashed look!

Wednesday 19th March 2003

Went to the gym this morning but did not feel too good so did not do a great deal. Tried some dresses on yesterday, got a lovely blue one from Kaleidoscope catalogue, a size 14 but tight (which is silly cos I can wear 12's now). Neil said it was lovely, one of the nicest dresses he has seen on me so I decided to keep it. I had sent for a gold one (in the sale) but it did not suit me. I have been looking on EBay for dresses and got the red one (on photos page) from the US. US sizes are different, so I am in a 12 here which is about an 8 there (I think?) though saying that when you look at their measurements I would go for a 10 in their sizes (very confusing!). One particular seller seems to sell a lot of stuff from a Charlotte Russe (never heard of her) but the stuff looks so sweet and romantic, so if you are in need of something different that is very flirty/romantic then do go look at this range (the sellers id to look for on EBay is vol_guy.). I think perhaps I should go out to the shops, but I am still reluctant to go try smaller things on (silly I know). It seems safer to get stuff online or from catalogues where I can try them on at home at my own leisure. I do rather like browsing on EBay, you can get some lovely stuff and so far everything I have bought has fitted (just!!). It's good to sell your old stuff on too (you know, all that stuff that is NOW too big for you!!) Click here to buy & sell on eBay! Here's the link to EBay!

Thursday 20th March 2003

R off school, J sent home from school (both sick....but recovering and driving me mad). A recipe for stress for me and already I have had some chocolate and nibbles several handfuls or sugary cereal. Now how much do I have to work on that railwalker tonight? I was going to be so good too.

Friday 21st March 2003

Does anyone need help on how to make dieting difficult for yourself?? I am very good at this really I am. Take today for instance. Started off well...good intentions...felt motivated...strong etc. Now, left the house this morning (to work in shop), Neil and J and R are all off sick, think Neil is the worst off, he feels awful and is in pain with his knee and back. Did a few hours in the shop (left early), stopped off at Woolworths and thought Mmmm why not get a few goodies for the kids and Neil, they need a treat. Bought some chocolate (ok a fair bit...ok a lot...well some of it was reduced in the sale). Got home, tired, hungry and in need of some instant energy. So opened chocolate and promised myself I would only have a bit....ate LOADS. Told the kids, who are still feeling pretty iffy...would they please eat the chocolate... PLEASE. Neil had some, though not a lot for him. THOUGH, knowing Neil he will work his way through it all by tonight. Why did I get all that chocolate?? Temptation on me and the kids and Neil certainly didn't need it. Well....no weight loss this coming week then. I am good at this aren't I.

I will definitely aim to go on the railwalker tonight. I am SO near to target and don't want to spend the next 6 months struggling to get there!!

Saturday 22nd March 2003

Got into a pair of jeans today that I have NEVER been able to get into, trouble is I bought them about 10 yrs ago and do not like the style of them now!!! Bought a load of grapes and every time I am tempted to pick... I go eat these (Ah is that why I have stomach ache now?)

Sunday 23rd March 2003

Managed to get through the night without picking¬ Now, today.....Too late to effect weight-loss for tomorrow, but there's next week. If I make it to the 8 st's tomorrow I am treating myself to a day out in Southport on Tuesday. I really really want to go to SPort for the day to toddle around the shops and meet Neil for lunch. I have not had a day out for ages. Now if I am not in the 8 st's??? What do I do?? Still go?? I will be good forever and ever and ever and give to all charities and never swear and be nice to everyone if I get into the 8st's tomorrow...really I will.

Slimming World Week 73

Monday 24th March 2003

Well...I will be so surprised if I have lost weight this week.

Slimming World Weigh-In
Weight = 9 st (126 lbs)
Stayed the same!
Total Lost So Far = 40 lbs
Lbs to go to target = 7 lbs

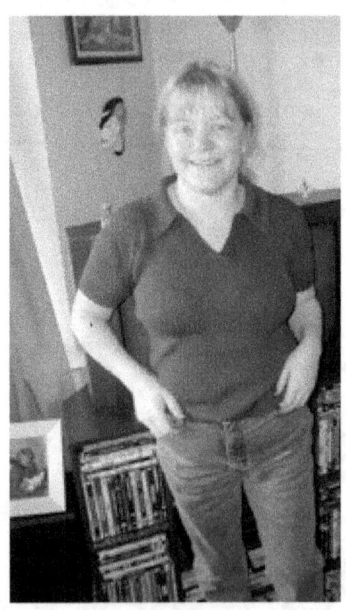

As you can see I have stayed the same, which is good. I have to admit I went back on the scales in the hope that they went to the 8st's, but they didn't, I was disappointed, quite a bit really, on the other hand I know I have not followed the plan 100% this last week. So...next week I WILL DO IT. I am going to Southport tomorrow and am going to have a nice wander round the shops (good, good walking!).I will not eat anything fattening, even when I meet Neil for lunch! We are having a meal out on Friday night (for J's birthday), but hopefully I can make good food choices and not hamper me losing weight this coming week.

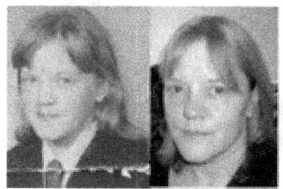

Here I am in 1974 age 12 and here I am in 2003 (today) age 39!!! Ah well. I am not falling apart yet!!!!!!

Have just eaten a HUGE bowl of leek and potato soup and am SO full up!

Tuesday 25th March

Went to Southport and walked and walked, my feet are killing me tonight (hope they recover by the line dance class tomorrow night! Got stopped for market research in Southport, the woman asked a few standard questions (where you from/what you do? etc) then said how old are you , I said 39, she was stumped for words (Hu? I thought?) then said can't use you, we only want to interview people age 32 and under, she said "you certainly don't look 39". Ha...that made my day I can tell you, being mistaken for 32 or less!!!!!! I do get so paranoid about looking older, having wrinkles etc. It's not that I won't grow old gracefully, but. well? Dunno??

Wednesday 26th March 2003

The scales, the scales they said 8 st 13 lbs!!!!!!!!! At the gym I had my fitness assessment and they said I was 8 st 13 lbs. I know I have to go by the Slimming World ones on a Monday, but to see an 8 st 13 is FANTASTIC. Did my yoga class....really cannot do the frog position but can do the crane/tree and other bendy bits and variations! It is linedancing class tonight, I am looking forward to it, it is nice to learn something new (now what about salsa?)! I think if I had the confidence I would love to do acting, I would enjoy this perhaps? Join some theatre group and have FUN and enjoy myself being someone else.

Really enjoyed the linedancing class and managed to stay for the 2 hours (2nd half is more difficult) and managed to join in the 2nd half without too many mistakes!! My feet seemed to know what they were doing even if my brain hadn't quite got the hang of it!!!!

Am feeling very determined and motivated

Ohhhhh have eaten so much spaghetti bol without the spaghetti that I cannot move, how on earth am I going to do in Linedancing in an hour.? I know it's best to eat the 'free' foods so you don't pick but I think I overdid it!

Sunday 30th March 2003

Well it was J's birthday on Friday, he was 12 and Neil's birthday on Saturday, he was 44. Mother's day today and poor old R (who is 5 with bday in Oct was feeling left out). Over did the snacky chocolate this last few days, although was very very good at the beginning and the middle of the week....but is this enough??

Slimming World Week 74

Have I made it into the 8 st's??

Monday 31st March 2003

I was good for most of last week and I did an awful lot of walking and some gym and a 2 hour line dance class - so let's hope this has done the trick and gotten me into the 8 st's!!! PLEASE. I know the gym scales said 8 st 13 lbs last Wednesday.......but obviously the days inbetween!!!!!!! Well... damage can be done unfortunately. It's about 20 minutes before I go get weighed and I am getting butterflies!! I want the scales to say 8 st something so much...and oh, I do hope they do. I certainly feel slimmer today!! A dress arrived from America that I have been waiting for ages and ages and I tried it on and it fits beautifully, will put photo up later). I am getting nervous.

Slimming World Weigh-In
Weight this week =8 st 13 lbs
(125 lbs)
Loss = 1 lb
Total Lost So Far = 41 lbs
Lbs left to go to target? = 6 lbs

YES I made it. I am now 8 st 13 lbs. I am so glad, I have not been in the 8st's since 1990 when I first met Neil.

Now I need to make sure I eat properly this week so I maintain this weight and even better, lose more!!

Tuesday 1st April 2003

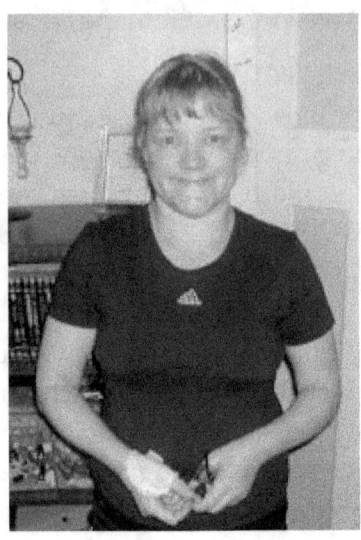

Ok here I am trying to look fit. Went to the gym and did an hour and then went for a tone and stretch class. Have discovered another room in the gym called the Torture Room!!! I really like the machines in there, hanging upside down or what!!! I did say to Kim "How do you get off this one?" Will go to the gym tomorrow and really work on those machines, they're great (ok, am saying this now, wait a few weeks!)Tonight Neil and I are going to my mum's 60th birthday meal (a surprise one). I cannot decide which dress to wear so will have a trying on session later.......am feeling in an un-fattish mood, so far!!

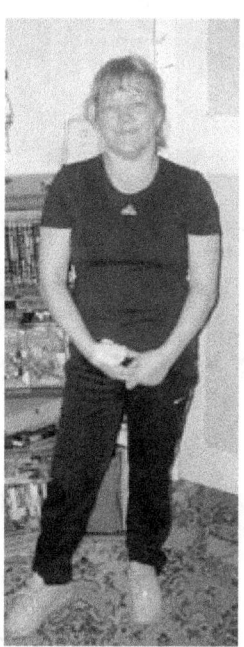

Bought this top from a sports shop cos it was in the sale, it never fitted, was far too tight (is double layered). Now it fits and is comfy.

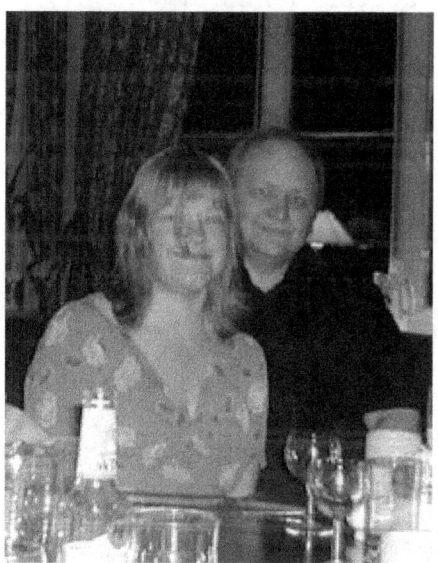

Here I am with Neil at my mums 60th birthday do.

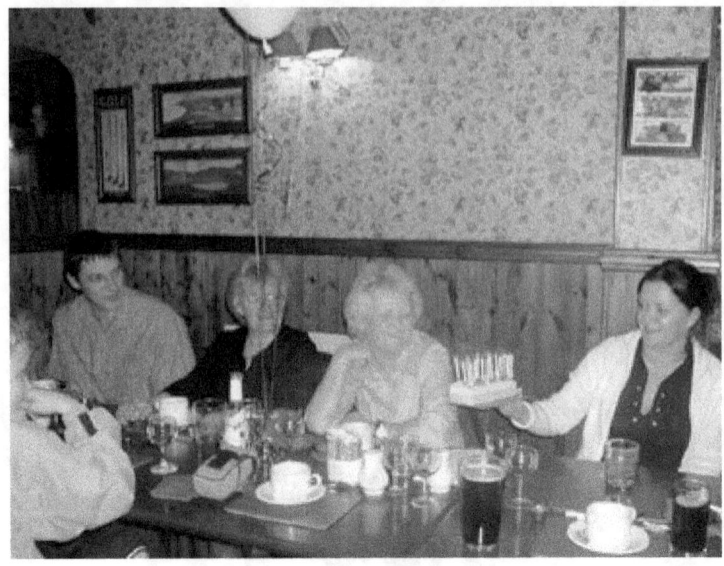

Then there's brother-in-law Peter, my sister Vanessa, my mum and other sister Cheryl (not in photo are my dad, other sister, nephew, Cheryl's boyfriend). We had a nice night, my 3 sisters were there and 2 of their partners and my nephew who is 13 (10 of us altogether for the meal).

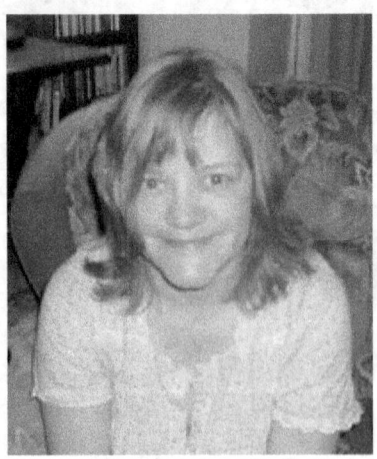

Here I am after the do, about to go to bed. It was a really nice night and a lovely meal (I did not over do it!!) And ok, I will work a little bit harder at the gym tomorrow. Neil enjoyed it too...he is not always comfy with family do's.

Wednesday 2nd April 2003

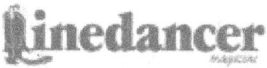

Off to my line dance class tonight (above is the logo of the LD mag - hubby works there!). Went to the gym today and did a yoga class. Am trying to correct those malteasers I ate last night on the way home from mum's do and the ermmmm 4 cookies I ate today!!! Seems so unfair how hard you have to work to work off the calories of just a few simple things (treats). I shall put a bit extra effort into the class tonight!! Had fun at the line dance class, really enjoyed it, though didn't seem to do so well with the steps this week. Am now going to try a Salsa class tomorrow night, have no idea what this will be like??

Thursday 3rd April 2003

Going to the gym today and the salsa class tonight. I should be sooooooooooo fit!!!! What do people wear to a salsa class?? Heels? Flirty dresses?? Jeans?? Arghhhhh I can see me flapping about this to night!! Am getting weighed in the gym this morning, I do not know how I might have done, but perhaps not so good as other weeks?? Well...mainly I go by the Slimming World scales on a Monday but when the gym ones show a gain it kind of gets you down a bit...or will make me be good the next few days!

Friday 4th April 2003

Well....I went along to the Salsa class (bit nervous as I went on my own). And I am sooooo glad I went, I really enjoyed it, it was great fun and not as difficult as you might think (although have only done 3 steps so far....mambo/side-step and susyQ I think that is what they were called!). I am going to do an 8 week course then can either do that 8 week beginners again or go onto the improvers!!

Friday 4th April Again

Have been very good today, even when I ate out at the cafe after working at the shop (I had a small latte and a brown bread ham sandwich). Then Neil got chips n stuff for the kids off the chippy and I never ate a one...not one (ok mainly cos there were none left by the time I got downstairs after being on the internet doing my poem to the music of Wouldn't It Be Loverly (My Fair Lady)....link on the front page). I have no idea how I might have done this week, I have certainly done more exercise this week. I had the meal out Tuesday night but did not overdo it apart from the bag of malteasers and have done my best not to nibble...though is difficult as there is a large pack of chocolate fairy cakes in the kitchen. So...Steve....I HOPE I do not see 9 st again.....we shall see and fingers crossed.

Sunday 6th April 2003

Well unfortunately I do think I have put on weight this week. I will be so fed up if I have gone back up to 9 st or over (worse still) but, I can feel it round my middle. I can feel the weight I have gained, except for when I am lying down! Then I feel slimmer (weird?). When I lie flat on the bed (is there another way?) I feel my hip bones/flatter stomach (where does it disappear to?) and I think Yeah Yeah...me slimmer ....BUT when I am standing it of course it still hangs there/wobbles there and my jeans are tighter (and they haven't been washed) and I think OMG I've gained some I have put a few lbs on I know I have. I cannot get away from the fact I ate ermmmmm a meal out/some malteasers/some matchmakers/other nibbles here and there and those I have forgotten about. SO......despite all the exercise I have done, I do think I have put on weight this week (boo hoo).

Slimming World Week 75

Monday 7th April 2003

Well...I am TOTALLY sure I have gained weight this week...so we shall see.

> Slimming World Weigh-In
> Weight= 8 st 13 lbs (125 lbs)
> Stayed the same!
> Lbs to go to target= 6 lbs

Oh mega! I have stayed the same weight, I am so pleased about this. I did not want to go back to 9 st anything, I think I would have felt really down had the scales said 9 something. Now if I lose (when I lose) a lb (or more) next week I will get my 3st award from SWorld. If anyone had said to me over a year ago that I would lose 3st (42 lbs) I would have said...no way. But, I've done it... I am almost at the weight I want to be... now Mmmm... let's keep it like that (like FOREVER!!)

Neil finally got weighed on Sunday and is now going to watch what he eats (hopefully), he weighed less than he thought (and me) he would because he ahs not weighed himself for ages. He is going to the Dr's on Wednesday (for his leg) and I am going with him, we are going to see about him going on Reductil. Ok it's 1 in the morning. I have had 10 sins today (that's ok). Have a lot of fruit in so will have this for brekky.

Ok, so this coming week I will be Sooooo Good!!

My friend Helen came round today, she joined Slimming World 4 weeks ago and has lost 8 lbs so far, which she is really pleased about. We sat and had a coffee and a chat (oooopppsss I offered her a biscuit! She said no). My other friend Judith (remember her?) well, she has put some on (won't say how much, or she'd go mad with me!). Judith, you need a holiday to motivate you....go book a summer one, then you can get losing for it!! I have counted the weeks, it is 16 weeks to our summer holiday in France...plenty of time for me to lose that 7 lbs or more and maintain!! Keep it off and tone up at the gym!!!!!

Tuesday 8th April 2003

Am collecting raffle money at my local hospital this morning, (Easter Egg Raffle).

Felt absolutely dreadful today and went to bed as soon as Neil got in. Hope I am feeling better tomorrow as I do want to go to the Linedance class.

Wednesday 9th April 2003

Made it to the linedance class though I did not do as well this week cos I felt so crappy. I may go to the gym tomorrow, feel as though I ought to. Neil went to the Dr's and we asked about him going on Reductil, though our GP prefers him to go on Zenical (I prefer he goes on Reductil)...anyway the GP said he has to lose about 7 lbs before he will consider him going on one of the drugs. So Neil is making an effort then will have to go back to the GP for a prescription.

Friday 11th April 2003

Why do I feel so fat this last few days? Even Neil commented on the size of my stomach, that was not nice was it?! I have been eating mints yesterday and some mini chocolate eggs (not so good) and feel yet again, I will not lose weight this coming week. To be honest, I can't be bothered this week, I haven't felt that good, have not been to the gym (though have done my 2 classes)...and I am fed up of having to think of what I am eating. I know perhaps I should not be so hard on myself, after all I have lost 40 lbs+ and feel so much better. But I so want to lose this last 6 lbs to target (and perhaps a bit more) and I am so close but well.....feels like it may as well be 60 lbs away. Ah well...hopefully I will feel better shortly?!

Saturday 12th April 2003

Took J and R and J's friends ice-skating today. J has never been before (nor me or R). , me and R were watching. J did ok, on his bum more than not at first! Then R wanted to have a go, so I hired skates for me and her. I have not been skating for 25 years! One of J's friends took R and took her round, she did so well and loved it. I never fell over once and even managed to pick up speed here and there and keep away from the barrier! It was good fun. I am glad I stayed on my feet as I thought, if I fall I will never get back up (easily anyway). We went to KFC and I had some food there (very fattening unfortunately) and despite me feeling yuck we had a Chinese last night (never ate that much though). Am hoping I (with J and R) might be able to go away for a few days with my parents and other family on a short break to Canaervon......dunno yet am waiting for mum to phone.

Sunday 13th April 2003

On the way home from my mums we stopped at Asda and got a pick and mix, now I feel yuck....serves me right! J is going away with my mum n dad (me and R are not) ah well. I cannot decided whether to go to Sw tomorrow or not, I really do not feel like going (I know I should go really), but I just feel like a week off from going. I know in truth that if I weigh myself in the morning and it says 8 st 10 lbs or thereabouts then I will go to SW. Silly I know. But I am soooooooofed up and annoyed with myself for eating badly this last week (and have used feeling crappy/sick as an excuse).

Slimming World Week 76

Monday 14th April 2003

Well how have I done this week? Have I held onto the 8 st's?? I hope so.

Found this site that does signatures, there are some very talented people doing them and they seem to do it for free. You can request anything and they get back to you so quickly.

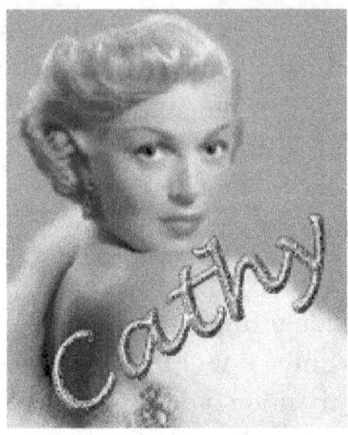

Slimming World Weigh-In
Weight = 8 st 13 lbs (125 lbs)
Stayed the same
Lbs to go to target = 6 lbs

Phew I stayed the same. I did go as you can see, I was not looking forward to it (kept thinking about all the stuff I have eaten this last week). I am going to be Sooooooooooo Sooooooo good this week.

I am glad I went to the meeting after all. I find lately, cos I am trying hard (ok not always so hard!) to get to target and it isn't far to go, well. Of course all my friends and family are pleased for me but I don't get the "Oh my god you've lost loads of weight" comments anymore. People who know me are used to how I look now and cannot remember how I looked a year ago. I find myself thinking 'Now who haven't I seen for ages (i.e. for a year or so!) and Mmmm maybe it would be nice to go visit them?' In fact I am wracking my brains to think of people whom I have not seen in a year...desperate to come up with people, anyone, long lost relatives!!! That's where going to meetings does help, they keep reminding you how well you have done/are doing and help you through rough spots. Close friends and family are perhaps bored now with it all? I think they will give a little cheer when I get to target, I hope they do anyway!!

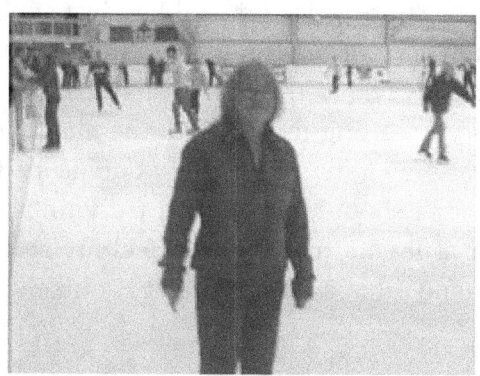

Here I am skating last Saturday, it was fun and I would definitely go again (if my joints are ok!)

Wednesday 16th April 2003

Went to Southport yesterday and did loads of walking (ok had an ice-cream too!). Today am in a FAT mood and nothing fits, everything I try on looks awful and it's beautifully sunny outside and because I am in a fat mood I don't want to go out, but then I don't want to stay in either. Dilemma! We have not had nice weather for ages and it is so hot out and I have rung everyone I know but most people have gone away for Easter. I think I might take R to the park later. Went to my friend Kim's, had lunch, then dropped R off at her nanna's then I went to Southport again (loads of walking here). It was very hot. This evening I managed to eat a load of profiteroles and some chocolate here and there....already I can feel it on my stomach. HELP I need to get back control of my eating. I have been overeating and it is so hard to stop!

Thursday 17th April 2003

Chocolate chocolate everywhere and it's not even quite Easter yet. And all I want to do is EAT. Am definitely in a hungry phase! Worse luck. And no exercise lately, though have done a lot of walking (my feet were FAR too knackered to go linedancing last night really they were). So... here I am, house full of other people's kids at the moment, desperate to go eat all in the cupboards and Neil had just spoken to me on aim to see did I want anything from the shops on his way home, or a takeaway. I said NO...NO...NO.

I have been scoffing myself with the mini eggs out of the cupboard, was only gonna have a few but ate loads, now I feel truly sick. Now I should be well and truly un-able to eat any chocolate for at least a month. I can feel my stomach, it is so HUGE. Neil and I have both got to get ourselves sorted out (diet wise)

Friday 18th April (Good Friday)

Went to get J from his nana's then we went on to Conwy North Wales. I had a banana split (yummy) that was my lunch. Then I had a cappuccino ice-cream (mega yummy), J did not want his so of course I could not throw it away. I was merrily walking along eating it when.....swooshhhhhhhh down swooped a blummin huge seagull and he nicked it from me. Took the whole thing right out of my hands. It was like a scene from Alfred Hitchcock's THE BIRDS. I screamed (albeit a few minutes later...the shock!). R then hastily gave me her ice-cream cos she did not want a seagull swooping down on her. I persuaded her to eat it (with my help) and her hand covering it (away from the birds sight).

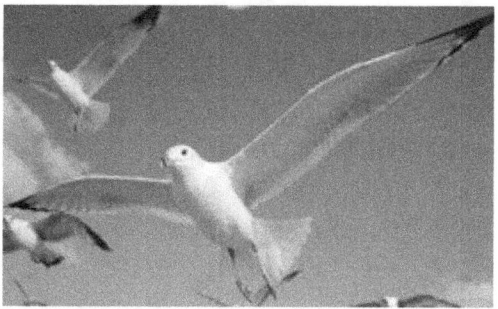

Perhaps the seagull KNEW I was on a diet and not supposed to have 2 ice-creams??

Saturday 19th April 2003

J and I are off on a day trip to Manchester (I will try to eat well...not much...carefully...very little...sensibly....as best I can....not too often....ah what the heck, it's a day out!)

Sunday 20th April 2003

Easter Sunday (Hope R and J eat all their eggs quickly... not leaving any in the fridge)

Slimming World Week 77

Easter Monday April 21st 2003

Happy Easter! Hopefully I have not been eating too many chocolate eggs!! Am not thinking too much about chocolate here am I? Did I really eat that much of it last week?

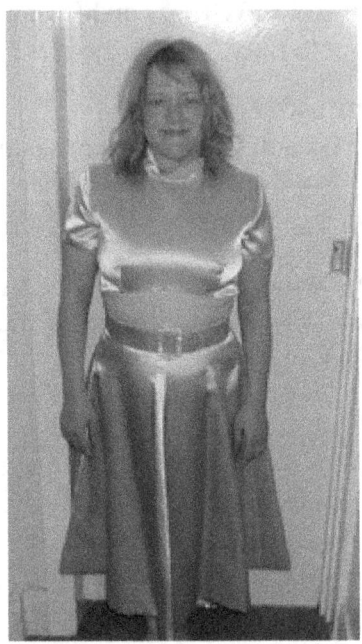

Here I am in a Grace Kelly Style dress that I got from the US (via EBay). This is the first time since I bought it, that it has zipped up (I was amazed). I have been trying it on for months and months.

Slimming World Weigh-In
Weight = 8 st 11 lbs
Loss = 2 lbs
Lbs to go to target = 4 lbs

Oh wow I have lost 2 lbs this week, I am now just 4 lbs away from my target (though I must be honest and say it feels more like about 14) I am so pleased though, and yes once again because I ate rather badly last week, I will have to eat properly this week. J and I went out delivering Slimming World leaflets yesterday, we were out for 3 hours (good exercise). Stacey is our new consultant and she starts next week.

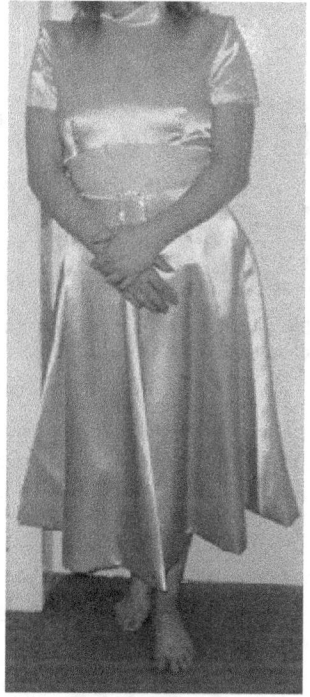

It really fits
I am ok...I have lost the urge for chocolate (really I have)!

Tuesday April 22nd 2003

Today R and I went to my cousins. I did ok the beginning of the day then I nibbled and ate chocolate on the way home.

Wednesday 23rd April 2003

Stayed in and tidied up (grrrr) but exercise, exercise. I think my eating badly will catch up with me this coming week. I Have to now keep relatively good control of my eating well...forever I guess. Not a permanent diet as such, but I will never have the kind of body that let's me eat what I want without gaining an ounce. Ah well.

Friday 25th April 2003

In the shop today. Did nothing in particular yesterday (but managed to eat about 6 kit-kats (WHY?). I am just being dumb now. Am I trying my BEST to put weight on, am I dilly dallying with the scales, am I messing about to see how far I can go???

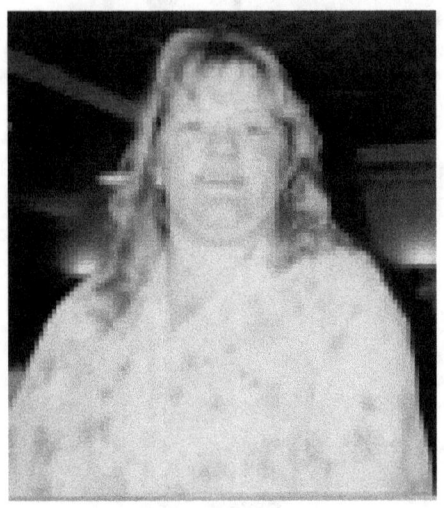

Just to remind myself WHY I should get back to eating properly

Sunday 27th April 2003

According to my scales I have gained about 2 and a half pounds....well...I must say I am not looking forward to getting weighed tomorrow. On the other hand it is a new consultant...so let's say A NEW START ok!! Neil, well, he is not doing so good, he has gained 4 lbs and he is trying to lose 7 lbs so he can go on Reductil. Perhaps if I have a new start now he can.

Slimming World Week 78

Monday 28th April 2003

I know... I just know I have gained weight this week... but how much? I want to get rid of this last weight, tone up a bit and be able to comfortably maintain my weight and keep it off especially by my summer holiday.

> Slimming World Weigh-In
> Weight = 8 st 11 lbs
> Stayed the same
> Lbs To Target = 4 lbs

Can you believe I actually stayed the same...the same weight. I can't! But I did. Body's are soooooo weird really they are.

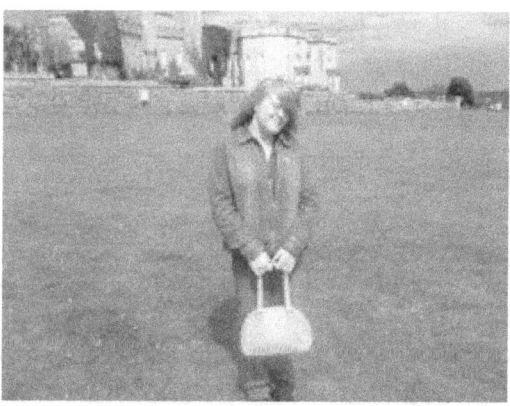

Here I am (and Neil and I) at Bodelwythan Castle North Wales on Saturday 26th April. We had a nice day out.

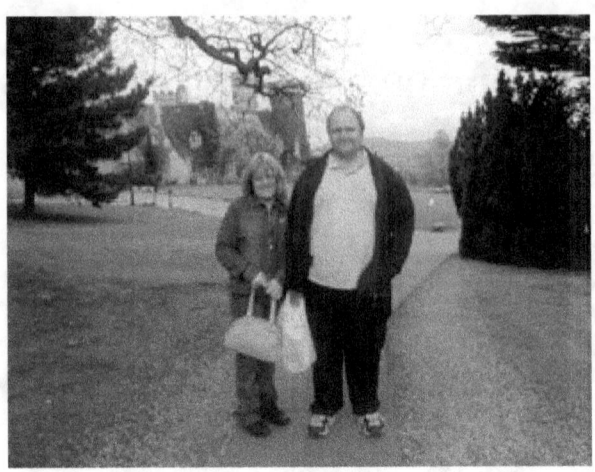

Neil is not happy with the way he looks on this photo. Last night I printed out a weeks sheet for us both to fill in...a food diary. We will do better.

Tuesday 29th April 2003

Spent the whole day in bed, when I woke up I could barely move, all my joints were hurting. I took double my anti-inflammatory dose and painkillers. Neil worked from home and looked after me. It is now just after midnight and I feel a little better, though still feel as though someone has stomped on my hands and knees. On the upside, I have eaten very little today.

Thursday 1st May 2003

Feel a bit better today. R is off school so we are having a lazy TV day. I am doing my best to eat properly, though half of me can't be bothered. Rang my sister, she said she stayed the same this week (she is doing SW too) but she will not tell me her weight or even her goal weight, still that is up to her.

Friday 2nd May 2003

Am in the shop today (am feeling sooo much better thanks goodness. It is one of the girl's birthdays in the shop and she has asked me to go for a coffee and some cake with her afterwards. Can't say no, will have to choose the one with the least sins, since I have already had over my sins allowance so far this week.

Sunday 4th May 2003

Ohhhhhhh why have I been soooooooooooooo bad? All week? WHY? Went to Warrington with Neil today, went to Ikea, had Swedish meatballs (YUM) and an ice-cream oh and ate almost a whole packet of mints (humbugs). Have not been exercising (not been well) so all in all a recipe for weight gain yes???? I think so.

Slimming World Week 79

Monday 5th May 2003

I certainly do have the feeling I have gained weight this week. I seem to be starting the weeks off ok....following the plan then going off it by the weekends, I am not doing it 100% and I think in order to get to my target I need to be more focused and eat better and make more of an effort. So...another week of a probable weight gain (am writing this Sunday night!). I have to have to have to make an effort. Neil has done well this week and lost 5 lbs. Unfortunately his eating this last few days has been awful, picking and cakes and sweets and things (ermmmmm bit like me really!)

Well I went along to Slimming World and got weighed and I got to target today. I really truly got to target, I am the weight I have been aiming for for 12 years. I am 8 st 7 lbs (119 lbs). I cannot believe it, I really can't. I actually lost 4 lbs this week (don't ask me how)??

Slimming World Weigh-In
Weight this week = 8 st 7 lbs (119 lbs)
Lost = 4 lbs (how????)
Total Lost So Far = 3 st 5 lbs (47 lbs)
Lbs to go to target = 0
(OMG!!!!!)I did it I got to my target weight!!

I am going to do a separate page of my fattest photos and lots of photos of me now (at target) so keep an eye on the menu page!!

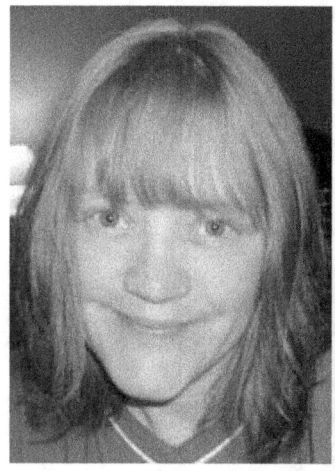 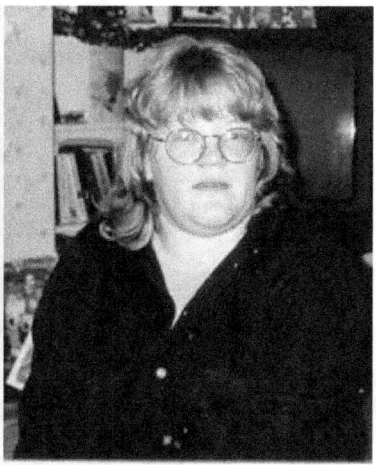

Here I am in the first photo taken 4th April 2003(age 39)at 8 st 7 lbs (119 lbs) and here I am in the 2nd photo taken about 1996 (age 31)or later (and I think I weighed about 12 st (168 lbs)

Tuesday 6th May 2003

Where do I go from here? Well... in truth I want to lose another 9 lbs (taking me to 7 st 12 lbs or 110 lbs), I think I will be happier at this weight and look better (especially round the middle. On the other hand if it proves very hard to get to or maintain, then perhaps I am better staying at the weight I am and toning up (if I can). I am only 5 ft and 7 st 12 would be a good weight for me, but I have not been this since I was 16. So......first things first, let me maintain this weight (knowing me I'll have a gain next week!), but that was my SW target 8 st 7 lbs (119 lbs) and here I am.

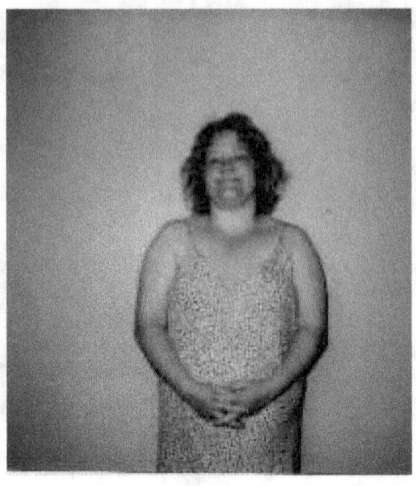

And here I was at 11 st 12 lbs (166 lbs)...big difference!! It's like now I have hit 119 lbs, I want less (to be less) to be less NOW, next week. But, as I have said not long ago, I have not been eating properly nor doing any exercise, so I need to get realistic and stop and go back to following the plan 100% and be more sensible and then, only then might I get an even lower weight.

Thursday 8th May 2003

Went to Southport yesterday and walked and walked ad walked (oh and shopped). Went to a cute Art Deco type cafe, very sweet, I was good and had a roast turkey sandwich (had ordered an egg one with came with mayo which I didn't want)..so there you go. Also went linedancing in the evening for 2 hours....that is why my feet are killing me today!

Saturday 10th May 2003

Feel fat...feel bloated, (must stop MOANING!). Must eat better, must go to gym more, must relax more, must chill out more, must stop picking, must get a job, must change the way I am, must stop being stupid, must stop ....what else? Did 15 mins on the railwalker tonight (it's a start back into exercise) I am aiming to go to the gym next Tue/Wed and Thur.

Slimming World Week 80

Monday 12th May 2003

I HATE my stomach, it is there, saggy and horrid. It is the only part of me that SPOILS me having lost the weight. Ok I can keep it held in with those type of knickers...I can hit the gym with a vengeance (joints allowing), I can lose another 10 lbs+ (which I want to do)...but will it ever look better?? I know it will never be flat, I am not aiming for flat but something that doesn't look like it's out of a horror film would be nice. Even Neil comments on it, he says he is joking but whatever...I HATE it, hate the way it looks/feels. I look AWFUL, a weird shape (when errrmmmm naked). I am not looking for perfection.....just a body that does not look so gross. I think I preferred my stomach when I was overweight, at least it was firm then!!! Ok gotta joke here or I'll get totally depressed.

> Slimming World Weigh-In
> Weight = 8st 8 lbs
> Gain = 1 lb
> Comments = I knew I had, but I am ok with it (soon get it off!)

Ok, so I have gained a lb this week, I felt I had and truly I know why I have (yes those sweets and chocolates I keep nibbling...fast, so they feel like they don't count but they do!). Took the Polaroid camera into class today to offer the use of it to anyone who wants a photo record of their weightloss journey. Have done a new page A Few Of My Favourite Things (might be boring for people, but I like it!! Well...at the moment!) Hey, I made it through the night without raiding the biscuit jar, I never had a nibble of a choccy biscuit....I am so glad and pleased.!!

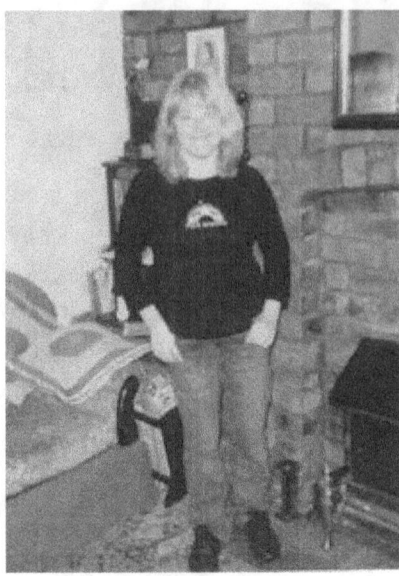

Me today!!!

Tuesday 13th May 2003

Went to the gym (first time in ages)...but my joints were hurting so I only stayed an hour and didn't do too much... will try again tomorrow. Was very good last night avoiding temptation, hope I can do it today! Neil has not been well (headaches etc). He did gain 3 lbs this week, but still, when you are not well. I am planning on going to the gym again tomorrow to do 2 classes.

Thursday 15th May 2003

Did my Linedancing class last night... hey I managed not to go wrong too much!! Neil is off work sick but eating...yes eating and making me eat too!!) Ha! I have never eaten so many grapes and free yoghurts in all my life. And have just had a huge bowl of scrambled egg (free) so how come I still...still crave the things I shouldn't have??? Huh????

Friday 16th May 2003

Here I am in a silver gown I got from the US, was very pleased that it fits (just)...but am fed up of things that 'just' fit and want them to fit perfectly...so come on Cathy get rid of this last 10 lbs (NOW)

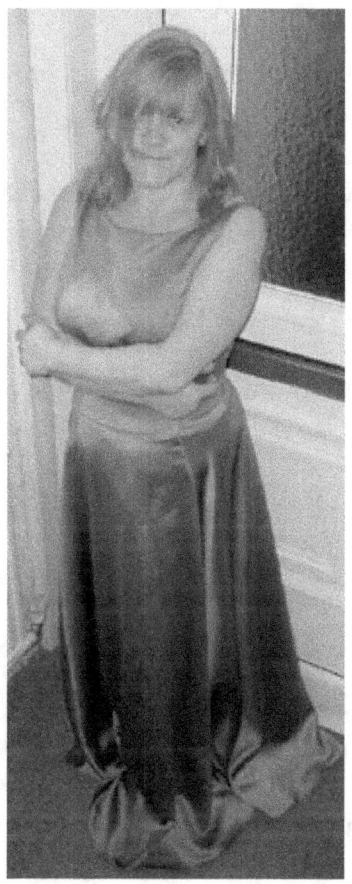

Sunday 18th May 2003

Managed to go to the gym this morning, did a legs/bums and tums class which was actually quite hard. It went very quickly, we did such a variety of exercises. Last night I did 15 mins on railwalker and am aiming to do the same tonight.

Slimming World Week 81

Monday 19th May 2003

Once again I know I have not eaten properly. Well, I seem to start the week off ok and stick to the plan but by the end of the week I have gone totally off it. I need a good week this coming week. I need to get back into good eating habits and to think twice about what I am eating. I am pleased with the fact that I went to the gym 3 times last week. Hopefully I will be able to get into a routine of exercise that I can manage.

Slimming World Weigh-In
Weight = 8 st 10 lbs
Gain = 2 lbs
Comments = Eeeeeekkkkk, have got to get back on track NOW

As you can see I gained 2 lbs, I knew I had I can feel it round my middle. So came away from the meeting with good intentions and will power. J is off school sick so we sat and watched Legally Blonde (and I ate grapes and ham - all free). Felt good. Neil came home early (sick) and later we had to go to Tesco...he said "I'm gonna treat myself" He does this a lot. He bought Donuts....on the way home in the car I ate almost 4 of them, one after another. WHY? WHY? I want to CRY.

Still, this is not gonna turn into a huge binge. I will count my sins (all 47 of them that I have had) and will do my damn best to be good for the rest of the week and put a bit extra effort into the exercise. But what a waste of sins, at the 3rd donut I was even feeling sick, but since I was in the car and there was nowhere to dump said donut, I carried on eating it and EVEN carried on pinching a bit of another one.

Wednesday 21st May 2003

Botheration. I have been eating badly again. How do I do it?? Had 4 biscuits today. Neil says he notices the part round my ribs is fatter (arhghghhg). Went to a meeting tonight and someone said "You've lost more weight haven't you?" (I took this to really mean "You are looking a bit chubbier") Have been wearing my 'fat' clothes, elasticated waists and baggy t-shirts. I must get a grip, get back on track and hopefully I will stop feeling so bloody tired and yuck.

Saturday 24th May 2003

Arghghghg. I have to get back to eating properly. Of course it does not help that my cooker has broken. At least I avoided takeaways this last week. I have now reached the point where I am looking totally flabby in my clothes. At the shop on Friday a woman said to me "how's the weightloss going?" (whilst pointedly looking at my expanding waistline. I mumbled about having got to target and relaxing a bit causing me to gain a few lbs. Well so far I have managed to gain 3 lbs but I know this is more, really I do.

How do I see myself?? I see me as FAT again, despite still being the lightest I have ever been and still under 9 st.

Slimming World Week 82

Wednesday 28th May 2003

Well, for the past few days I have been in my parents house with the kids. The kids are off school for half term and I took them there for a mini break. You can never eat as you want in other people's houses...and I did eat a fair bit of chocolate in my sisters! Today I am off to my sister-in-laws (it is her sons birthday) ok MORE food on offer. What I will do is aim to eat the less fattening stuff OK!

Ok so I had some teeny weeny pieces of pizza and the odd chocolate roll and some strawberry cake (oh it was so yummy), but other than that I was good!! Now.....tomorrow I WILL follow the plan, I will chill out (Thanks Siobhan for your message in the Guestbook... I will enjoy my new weight). I know I need to start eating better again (so I don't pile on the lbs) but as Siobhan says, a few pounds on at the moment, compared to all I have lost is nothing.

Didn't get weighed this week as I was away.

Went Linedancing tonight and my feet are throbbing!! But I enjoyed the exercise.

Thursday 29th May 2003

Parents came down to help with flood under floorboards. Later on was driven to shop and made to feel better with the aid of malteasers! Now feel sick. And fat. I feel sick and fat (just what I need). I will have a better day tomorrow. I will.

What was I saying about today??? Yes today Friday 30th May 2003

Well... still some water under floorboards. Drains people came/jetted/camera down there and quote of £2080.00 GULP. Finished off chocolate matchmakers and malteasers for comfort. Felt sick then ate nothing else all day. Managed packet of crisps and grapes and yoghurt. Feel sick again. Is this stress?? It is hard to concentrate on oneself when the house is in chaos.

Saturday 31st May 2003

It is round about 9 weeks to our summer holiday in France. Now... I am aiming to lose about 10 lbs or so before the holiday (let's see what I weigh on Monday first!!)...I need to make an effort. So we are staying near Benodet. I am really looking forward to it. Last year when we went to France I weighed 10 st (140 lbs). Last weigh-in I was 8 st 10 lbs (122 lbs....so already am (was?) 18 lbs less than last years holiday at the moment). I would like to be 7 st 12 for this coming holiday (110 lbs). So I gotta make an effort. So if I do it (when I do it) I would be 30 lbs lighter than last years hol FANTASTIC. I have got to got to do it.

Sunday 1st June 2003

Neil got weighed this morning and has gained a lb. I have probably done the same or more. Will get weighed tomorrow at Slimming World. Perhaps it will not be so bad as I think?

Slimming World Week 83

Monday 2nd June 2003

Ok... so how have I done? It is about time I got back on track isn't it. It is easy to think "Oh now I have lost the weight, no need to diet, no need to make an effort or watch what I eat". But I know this is NOT the thing to do.

> Slimming World Weigh-In
> Today I weigh = 8 st 7 lbs (119 lbs)
> Lbs lost so far = 47 lbs
> Now I want to lose about 7+ more lbs
> (and hopefully I'll be happy!)

Oh my goodness I have lost 3 lbs (dunno how exactly). So I am back at my current target weigh. Today was a good meeting at Slimming World even though there were not many people there. I feel I am now able to get back on track and stick to the plan. I have not really been following the plan properly this last month or so and although I have lost weight and gotten to my target, I think it has been more as a result of not eating properly (and perhaps high blood sugars) rather than sticking to the SW plan. It is very important for my health that I get back to eating properly, not doing silly things like missing meals here and there or my meal consisting of being a big bag of sweets!

Am feeling good and motivated and DETERMINED

Wednesday 4th June 2003

Have not been very well (joints are hurting and feel like crap). Am eating... well, mainly just pieces of bread and butter, that's all I feel like eating at the moment. Went to rheumatologist yesterday who put up my MTX to 25 mg. I do like my in-laws scales, on them it says I am 8 st 4 lbs (116 lbs)....I still find it weird to step on the scales and the number does not shoot up to 11 st something (145 lbs+). I keep expecting the dial to go up further and ever so briefly and baffled as to why it doesn't! (Silly eh!!?)

Thursday 5th June 2003

Been messing around with Photoshop! These were taken today.

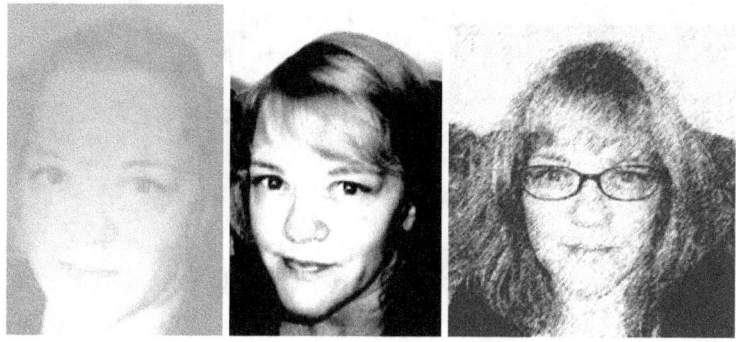

I am going to make an effort and really stick to the plan. I feel a bit better today, not so yuck. This is what I am wearing today.

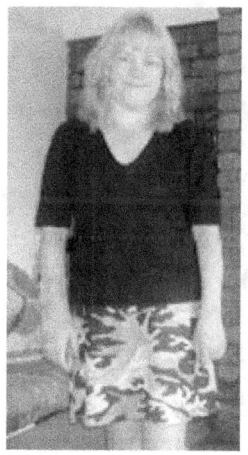

I am feeling in a slim mood (he he so far). Thank you Kathy (My best friend in Ohio), she said I looked skinny!!!!

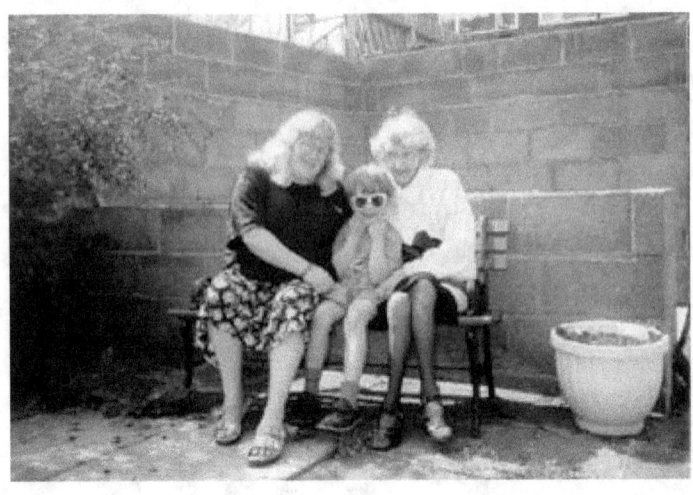

Here I am in 1995 (or was it 96?) with my Auntie Nellie (she died 2 months after this photo was taken). I really miss her. She knew me (of course) when I was thinner and didn't like the way I had become (fatter) after having J. I think she found my 'fatness' hard to deal with and I am truly sorry she never got to see me reach my goal (target weight). I am sure she would have been proud of all the weight I have lost.

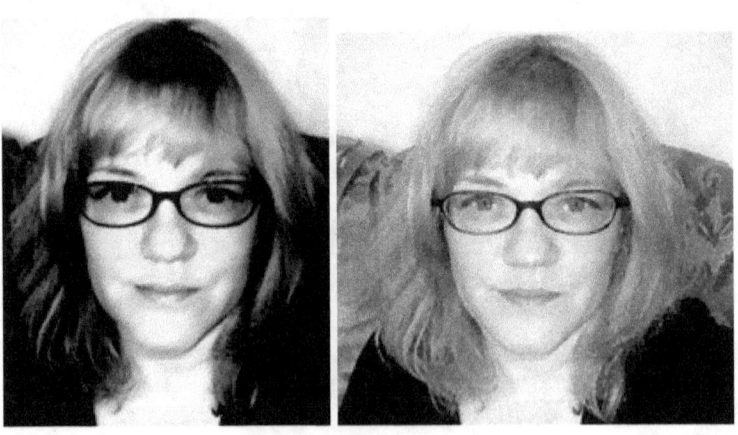

Same photo, taken today 5th June 2003. Mainly I wear my glasses every day (saving my contact lenses for special occasions). On the other hand I take my glasses off when I am having my photo taken. I like wearing glasses but it is nice to have the contacts for a change.

Ok....lose 47 lbs, get some new clothes (good idea)....lose 47 lbs and book a holiday (fab idea)....lose 47 lbs...treat yourself to a few new things (great)....lose 47 lbs and dye your hair bright RED (ermmm....dunno, have only just done it, it is evening and have not seen it in daylight yet.) My daughter thinks it's not real hair. My son doesn't know if he wants to be seen with me (he's 12). It will probably clash with loads of clothes! It IS permanent. It is bright. I saw the hair dye in Tesco and thought (wow love that colour) and well...there you go and here it is?

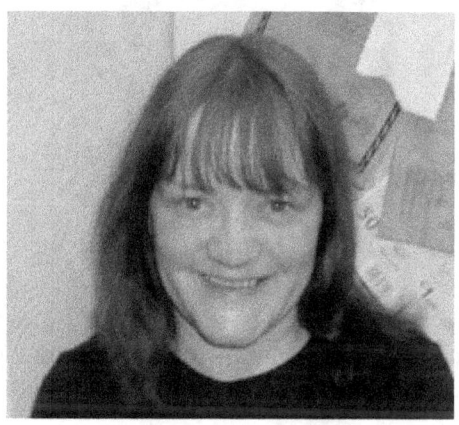

Here I am with my newly dyed hair (on a whim) and well.....I do like it (gotta say that) but have not been out in public with it yet) It is almost 10.30 at night on Friday 6th June and I have not long done it like this. Have emailed loads of friends for their opinions...............what do you think?

Saturday 7th June 2003

Lovely and hot today. The hair saga...well, hair is now darker, liked the bright red but couldn't handle the stares at the supermarket! So hair is now a darker shade of red. perhaps this was not the right time of year to do it? I hope it does not go green in the swimming pool when on holiday at beginning of August!! We went to WK marine lake today (I fancied chips but only ate a few)...Neil ate loads, then we got on to discussing his weight and how unhappy he is with it. So, our holiday is in 8 weeks and he can lose a lot in that time if he makes an effort. And I still want to lose another 10 lbs....so from tomorrow we are both going to stick to the SW plan and help each other. We will do it.

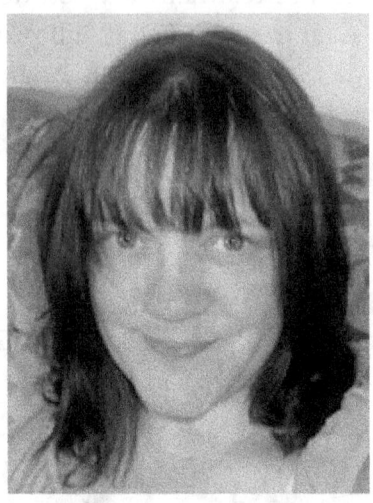

Mmmmmm just how many colours can I go in a short space of time?

Sunday 8th June 2003

It's still the same colour!!!! Neil got weighed and is 19 st 2 lbs (or 268 lbs and a bit). Today we are BOTH going to follow the SW plan and keep to it ALL week. It will be hard for Neil, he does have such a big appetite and there are so many foods he does not like (mainly veggies and salads). His diet has always consisted of bread (more bread) meat and roast potatoes (no other) and the usual cakes/ sweets/ takeaways/ crisps/ more cakes/ more bread. He will eat fruit now (limited to strawberries/apples and pears). And he likes Muller yogs (I rely on these so much). So... he will have mainly red days (Original) and hopefully we will get that weight off. He was going to be able to go on Reductil but his blood pressure is so up (even with tablets) that NO way will our GP now give him the Reductil. I know he is VERY unhappy with the way he feels and looks, and if I am truly honest I think he looks awful too (sorry Neil) . I know that he can do it, he has lost weight in the past (many years ago, he got down to 16 st and when I met him he was between 13 st and 14 st).......so this time he will do it. I know he finds the fact that it is so much to lose a bit of a mountain and cannot see an end in sight, but it took me a year and a half to lose 3 and a half stone and if anyone had said it would take that long at the beginning, I would have given up I am sure. Neil is determined and I know I need to help him as much as I can.

Slimming World Week 84

Monday 9th June 2003

Think I may have had a little gain, but still. Yesterday I actually stuck to the plan as did Neil. We ARE going to have a good week. I have been trying on clothes cos the local branch of our Diabetic group is having a 'Do' on Friday 20th June, loads will be there including all the Consultants. What do I wear? Don't want to be too dressed up on the other hand it will be nice to dress up (a I never go anywhere to get dressed up for). Get weighed later....fingers crossed!

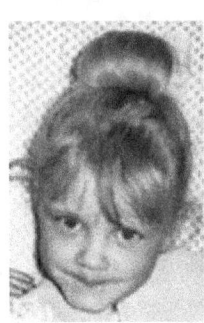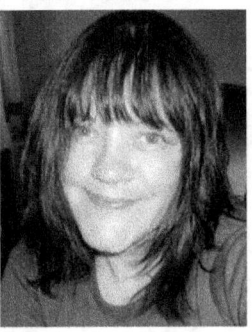

Here I am age 4. And here I am (right) age almost 40!!!! Talk about changed from when I was fatter!!!!!!

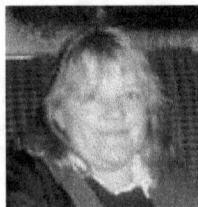

Here I am about 2 yrs ago

Slimming World Weigh-In
Weight this week = 8 st 7 lbs
Stayed the same
Total Lost = 47 lbs

I enjoyed Slimming World class and was pleased to have stayed the same.

Neil and I had a good day yesterday.

I want to lose about 10 more lbs by 1st August.

Wednesday 11th June 2003

Have been fairly good the last few days, but did have a few too many little choccy bikkies last night (gave in at last minute). Still, there is the rest of the week to make up for it. Neil is managing to stick to the plan but is hungry (missing his snacks). Have been trying on clothes again and am disgusted with stomach. Have bought holderinnerknickers which make it look slightly better but feel annoyed cos they are SO nylon. Bras are a pain too, some I pop out of, some are too big and hold up nothing. Ermmm perhaps I ought to go for a fitting? At some point I might. I am paranoid cos I have one breast bigger than the other and I soooooooo notice it and I hate it, try to squash it down but this does not work and try to lean forward with right shoulder to 'displace' them almost, so they look even, but they don't.. So here I am (moaning again) have one boob that sticks out more than the other, have lumpy tummy that looks like lumps of sculptures clay (un smoothed)......hair colour that keeps washing away (so will eventually be PINK) and ermmm what else? Think that's about it for the moment.

Thursday 12th June 2003

Enjoyed my Line Dancing class last night. Good exercise and fun. Got my new SW steamer out of the box (at last) and am now steaming some yummy veggies for later).I am determined to lose some weight this week. At my Line dancing class last night a woman came up to me and said "Cathy, you are wasting away" Ohhh I was so pleased to hear this!!!! Sometimes it depends on what you are wearing. Yesterday I had on a red t-shirt and a pair of jeans which are loose on me. With the weather being sunny too, I am not wearing a big coat/jacket that usually covers me up. I bought a mag yesterday, I thought it was on diet but it was a plastic surgery special, Some woman had the same stomach as me (yep!) and was my height and weighed a few lbs less than me.......and had a tummy tuck. She looked fab. I WANT ONE (a tummy tuck) but it is sooooo expensive (between £2,500 and £5,800)

Friday 13th June 2003

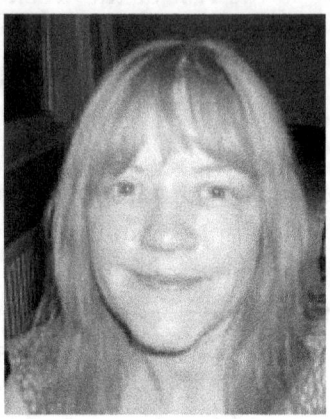

Ok...OK...I have gone back to my normalish hair colour. It has the odd bit of pink in it here and there but is more or less how it used to be. I wasn't 100% happy with it dark. Sometimes I liked it, sometimes I didn't. Don't think I have ever been so many colours in so few days! Cost a fortune. I got the feeling not that many people liked it dark, not that that terribly matters...but I found myself wanting it blonde again (hehe for now!!)

Saturday 14th June 2003

Neil got weighed this morning and he has lost 7 lbs. That is so great, I am really proud of him. He has been sticking to the Slimming World Plan all week and followed it well. He said that after a while he never felt as hungry. He has mainly the Original (Red) days though I shall try him on the Green days too for some variety. He is now in the 18 st's (Gone down into the next stone).

Slimming World Week 85

Monday 16th June 2003

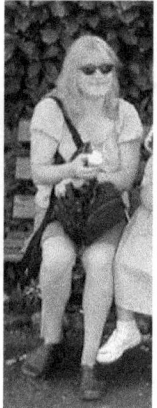 Am off to Chester Zoo today (helping my little girl's class) so I won't be getting weighed in the morning, but I am thinking of going to the evening class (even though I will weigh a possible 2 lbs heavier!) I have just got to get weighed! I did have an ice-cream (as you can see!), it was soooooo hot, we also did quite a lot of walking.

Monday 16th June 2003

I did go and get weighed and had gained a lb, which is ok.

> Slimming World Weigh-In
> Weight this week = 8 st 8 lbs
> I gained a lb, but that is ok since I got weighed in the evening (not my usual morning).

Went to my mums on Sunday and they had a buffet, I was okish, had loads of salad but all the sandwiches were made with white bread which is 'sinned' on the slimming world plan.

Wednesday 18th June 2003

Ok, I had a small pack of biscuits I never meant to eat. My feet are killing me, I went to Southport yesterday (walked for ages) and tonight I could not go to my Line Dance class (no way).

I bought a body fat calculator from Avon. The sort you hold in your hand (after keying in your weight/height/age/sex) It said I was 23.8 % body fat. The range for me is 20 to 27 %....so I am doing ok!!. Neil's said 38 %, well over his range.

Slimming World Week 86

These weeks go on forever!

Monday 23rd June 2003

How have I done? Well I ate badly the last week, nibbling lots. Had the DUK branch anniversary buffet and have done very little walking cos my joints have been bad...so am expecting some gain.

Saturday I bought some holiday clothes and was pleased to have gotten into these size 10 shorts easily.

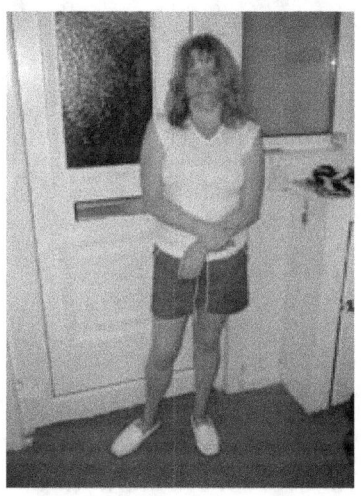

Slimming World Weigh-In
Weight this week = 8 st 5 lbs or 117 lbs
Loss = 3 lbs
Total Lost So Far = 49 lbs
I want to lose 6 more lbs before my holiday at the beginning of August.

Went and got weighed and was surprised to have lost 3 lbs. Perhaps I stick to the plan far more than I realise? I certainly do eat less than I used to, it is more a good habit now.

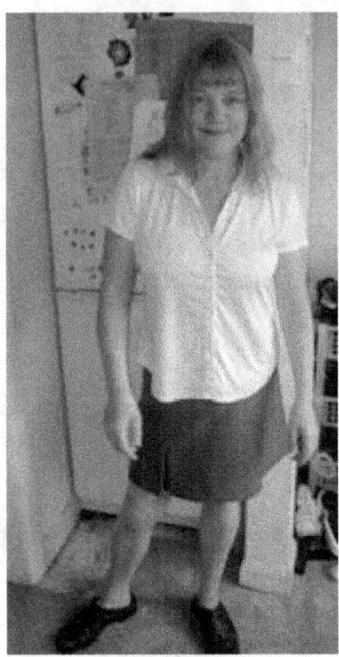

Summer holidays
HERE I COME !

Am feeling very positive about losing the last of my weight, even if I do have a small gain next week. Have been trying to telephone everyone I know to tell them I got my 3 and a half stone award, but like a thing on purpose, everyone is out!!

Tuesday 24th June 2003

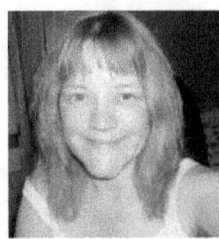

I have really been sticking to the plan and feel good abut myself. The weather was hot and sunny today and I did a bit of sunbathing...ok, I still look as white as ever, maybe a bit pinker! Today I wore some beige trousers (arghghghg beige!) and a white top and felt I looked ok, slim even!!

There's a first, little by little I am getting used to the new me and realising I am not FAT. Helps that today was not a 'fat' day as such, you know one of those days where you get out everything in your wardrobe and you look HUGE in it all, everything.

This is the first summer I can feel good about myself.......so let's have some great sunny days please!

Wednesday 25th June 2003

Not that I use the phone much...do I Neil? Helped out at the school sports day today, it was so hot. Tonight I went to my Line Dancing class and now my feet are so aching! Afterwards I did give in and eat a handful of biscuits (well to be exact 6 rich tea ones and about 6 choccy ones)..wish I hadn't now, still not a binge as such so I have the rest of the week to be good.

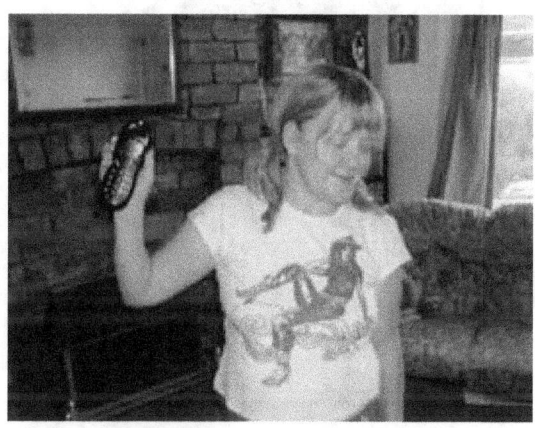

Before linedancing class

Saturday 28th June 2003

I helped out at the school fair today, it was fun. I never ate a thing (despite being right next to the bar-b-q. Then at the end of the fair the cake stall had loads of cakes left and it was such a shame to see them go to waste (since parents had baked them) so I bought some (ok lots). Got home and scoffed at least 8 of them (they were small cakes). Wish I hadn't!!! Tomorrow I am on a canal boat trip with J (and some other people), we get to have dinner at a pub and take along some wine?!

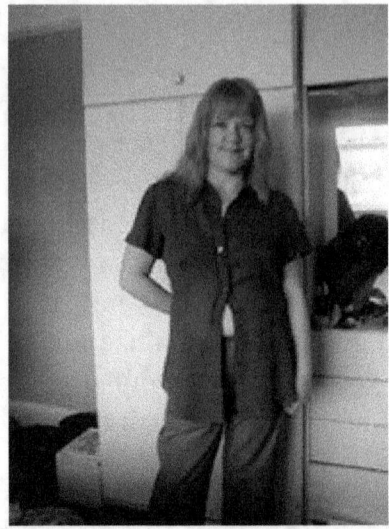

Me before the school fair

Slimming World Week 87

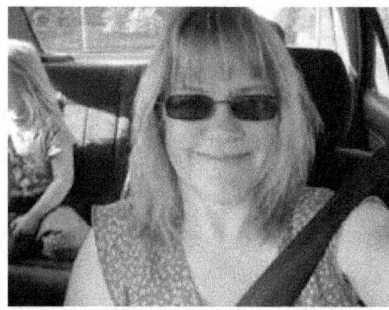 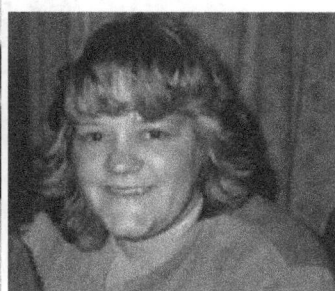

1st photo was taken yesterday and this 2nd was taken 1997
(when I weighed about 30-40 lbs heavier.)

Monday 30th June 2003

I have almost certainly gained weight this week because I have not eaten so well. I have picked a lot and eaten loads I never meant to. If I want to get rid of these last lbs for my holiday I need to make an effort and stick to the SW plan 100%. I know I CAN do it. I have been looking round all the shops for the 'perfect' swimming costume and have not found it!!!! I have been searching on eBay and seen a wonderful 1960's blue one with 2 daisies on it....I would rather like to win it. Also I have ordered a red one piece from La Redoute....in a size 10 (That's a US 6/8 I think).

> Slimming World Weigh-In
> Weight this week = 8 st 6 lbs (118 lbs)
> Gain = 1 lb
> Total Lost So Far = 46 lbs
> Lbs left to lose? = 8 ish

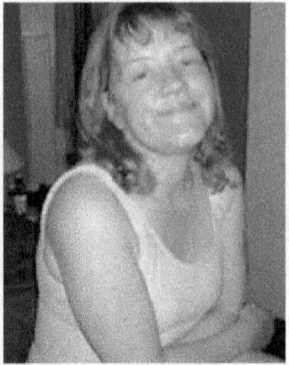

In my blue swimsuit, I feel I look ok but need to lose about 10 lbs. Also I have been trying on my 2 bikinis and I would wear them on holiday as I look now but would prefer to be a bit less flabby

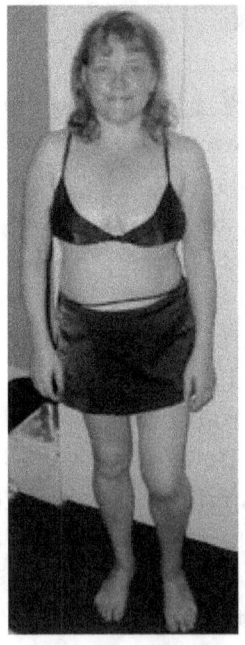

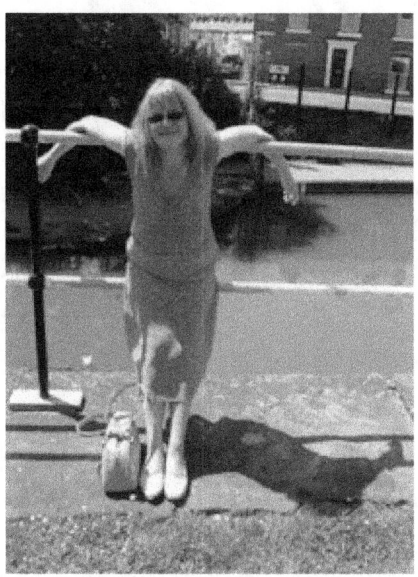

Here I was yesterday on our canal boat trip. It was so hot and lovely and we all had a brilliant time. In the pub I had a chicken salad!

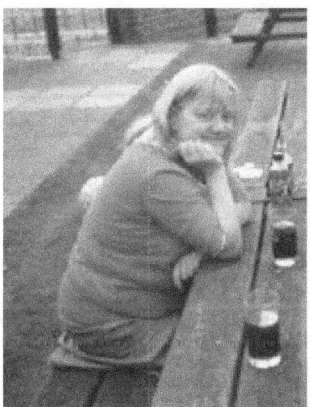

On holiday last year, where I felt slimmer and was about 10 st (140 lbs). This yrs holiday I am hoping to weigh about 110 lbs or thereabouts and at the moment as you can see I weigh 118 lbs.....so just 8 lbs to lose. Some people might think 'Oh why is she going on about losing 8 lbs more'? But it's something I want to do and will do (I hope)!I want to feel good on my hols!!!

Wednesday 2nd July 2003

My knee has suddenly become swollen and I can hardly move it. It is not terribly painful, just awkward to move. I am taking my anti-inflammatory tabs and painkillers, hopefully it will settle down soon. Scoffed a few choccy biscuits in sympathy with myself yesterday, oh and today (naughty). Now I feel flabby, but lying on the couch makes you feel like this too..

Slimming World Week 88

After my weekend away!

Monday 7th July 2003

Slimming World Weigh-In
Weight this week = 8 st 10 lbs (122 lbs)
Gain = 4 lbs
Lbs I want to lose before holiday = 10

I have been away for the weekend. The weekend started off on the Friday morning and lasted till Sunday night!!! As you can see I actually gained 4 lbs this week, the most I have gained for quite a time. I ate much more than I normally would while away but had been not so good before I went away also... so there you have my 4 lbs. I started off not really paying much attention to what I was eating then by Sunday I was being more careful. Though I did have my fair share of alcohol, which I don't normally drink. It was a lovely weekend (a diabetes related training weekend). There were a lot of nice people on it and it was tiring/intense but fun.

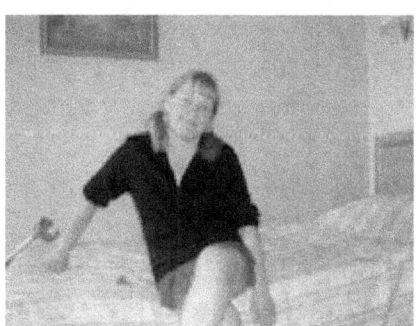

Here I am sitting in my hotel room

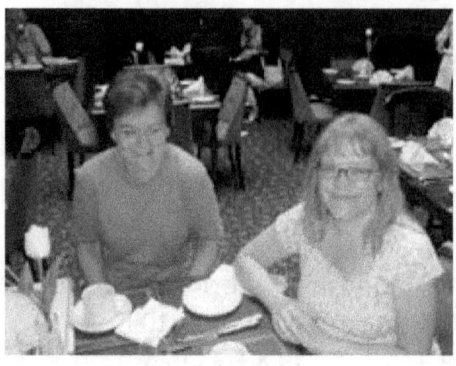

Here I am at the hotel (eating!), we seemed to eat a lot (often). I expected to have a gain and I am pleased that I am still within my target range (just). So today I am back on track and will get losing again. I had a lovely weekend and did not stress or worry about what I would or would not eat, I think I was sensible and did not go on a 'binge' and whilst 4 lbs might seem like a lot...I feel it is ok (ok, perhaps if this had taken me over my target range I might not feel quite like this!!!)

Thursday 10th July 2003

Well, tomorrow I am going to my local college for an interview/info appointment so I may do a 1 yr course in September to brush up my office skills and gain some current pieces of paper (qualifications). I have thought about doing this for a few years now but never got round to actually going for it, so now I am.. It's about time I did something. Ok, I am working at Oxfam and helping at school, but I need a paid job and I need a change. I have done office work in the past and I met Neil when I was doing an office admin course in 1990. I feel 99% happier with how I look and DO feel more confident... So, am looking forward to updating skills. Have just bought 2 packets (buy 1 get 1 free) of kit-kats and I soooooo have to not eat them! Got them for the kids (seeing as R is having a friend home to tea).. I will do my VERY best not to go eat any of the kit kats especially since I am trying to keep my blood sugars lower (besides wanting to lose some weight this week!

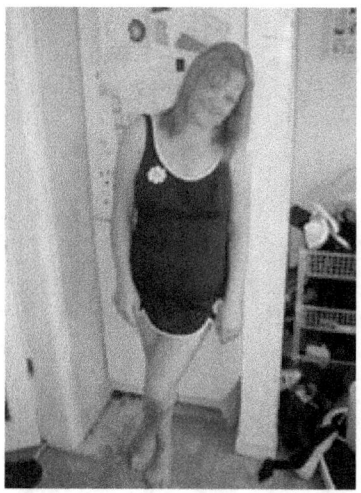

Here I am in my super daisy swimsuit (a la 60's style or thereabouts!) It is so cute (the swimsuit not me!) and I really like it.

Friday 11th July 2003

Had my interview today at the local college. Am now I am going to do a 1 year course there starting in September. I am so glad I applied and even more glad I got on the course, I am really looking forward to it, I am sure I shall really enjoy it and....well, as is the purpose of it....get a job I will enjoy after I have done the course.

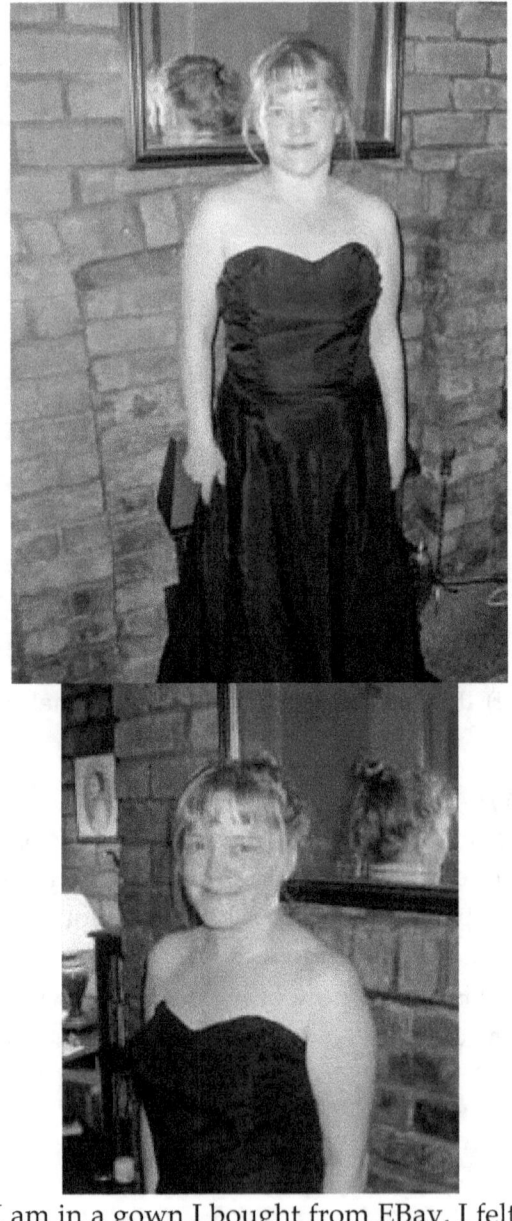

Here I am in a gown I bought from EBay, I felt like trying it on, it fits fine but is far too long so I need it altered. I wonder if I will ever get the chance to wear it (on an occasion)? I don't suppose so.. It has a little short sleeved bolero jacket that goes with it which is nice.

Saturday 12th July 2003

Went to my mums with the kids for the day. Spent the day in the garden sunbathing and am now peeling (oh bugger), was trying to get a bit of colour before we go to France in just under 3 weeks...but have managed to give myself a red stripe across my tummy. For some reason I figured, if I get some colour on my middle (the flabby bit) well, it won't look so flabby? But it still looks flabby and crappy and now is bright red (and hot) also. It was lovely being out in the sun, had a choc-ice!!! We ate on the way home at the OK Diner and I avoided a dessert!

Slimming World Week 89...
yes 89, that many

Monday 14th July 2003

Can you believe it is less than 3 weeks to our holiday in France.

I really think I have gained weight this week, again. I have not followed the plan properly and feel very bloated so I am not terribly looking forward to getting weighed. But I will get weighed and I will NOW stick to the plan, I have 2 weigh-ins left till we go on holiday. I am pleased to say I have lost a lb this week, this is such a motivator for the rest of the week. Today I am having an 'original' day and am just about to go eat some sin free sausages with loads (and I mean loads) of peppers/onions and tomatoes - yummy.

Slimming World Weigh-In
Weight this week= 8 st 9 lbs
(121 lbs)
Loss= 1 lb
Lbs I want to lose = 9 lbs+

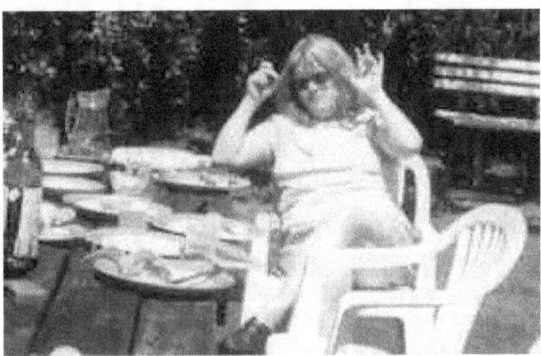

Here I am on holiday in France last year (July 16th 2002) - I weighed 10 st (140 lbs).

Tuesday 15th July 2003

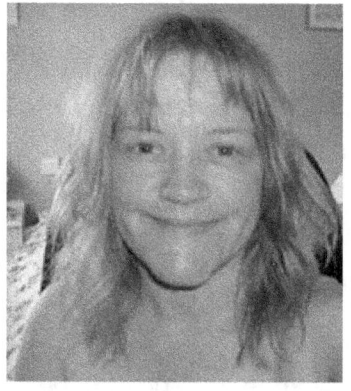

Gosh it is sooooo hot. My sister came down and we went shopping for holiday t-shirts. Got a cute strappy pink one. Made the mistake of buying mint choccy biscuits and putting them in the fridge - they are freezing and YUMMY and have had 3 already today (so no sins left). Was so good otherwise and had got myself a fantastic mixed salad for lunch.

Friday 18th July 2003

Seem to have 'picked' a lot this week. Got invited to a school 'thank you' tea this afternoon and had a scone (2 of them) with cream). Have been nibbling Everton mints and a biscuit here and there. What started out as an ok week has quickly gotten worse. I must admit I do feel very fat round my middle...not good. I was hoping to have lost some this week and the next ready for my holiday...but I know I have gained. I am going to aim to be good the next few days and then onwards till we go on holiday (2 weeks time).

Slimming World Week 90

Monday 21st July 2003

I have a feeling I will have gained this week...no matter. I will have a VERY GOOD week this coming week for my last weigh-in before my holiday. On Saturday we went for a walk round WK lake and had 2 (yes 2) ice-creams...one at the start of the lake and one at the other end. Ok so here I am in another 3 bikini's I bought (the sort that holds in your tummy!). I don't think I look that good (hey perhaps it's the bikini's not me?) and I wish I could change my body shape (n get rid of tummy and other annoying bits).

> Slimming World Weigh-In
> Weight this week = 8 st 10 lbs
> Gain = 1 lbs
> Lbs to lose = about 10

I went to SWorld and got weighed and had gained a lb and yesterday I already started writing down all I am eating, I am going to follow the plan to the letter. I AM going to have a good week. Ok, I admit it I ate 3 (I think it was 3) chocolate biscuits today, but I have counted them (reluctantly)..but counted them all the same.

Still wish my tummy was flatter but perhaps I am not quite so self conscious of it now (I am getting used to it!) I do feel that by losing another 10 lbs+ then I will feel even better and I WILL do it (but perhaps realistically it will be after the holiday... we go on the 1st Aug. Have just been reading a short article about how much you can lose in 2 weeks if you really try...so I am gonna try!

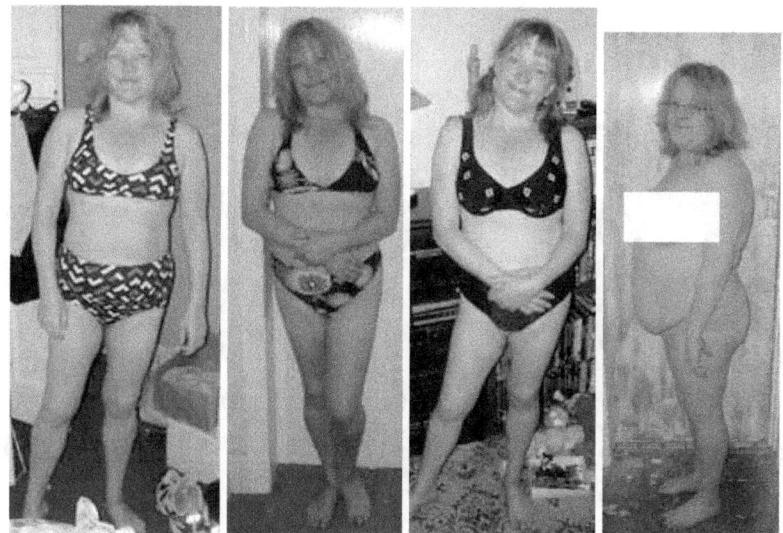

So here are the bikini's for my hol and whilst I am not 100% happy with how I look...compared to how I looked in 2001 (4th photo)......well what the hell am I whinging about!!!!!!!

I am really going to do my best, I have 11 days to go till the holiday. I have been having a go on the railwalker, though have to be careful as my knees are being a bit funny (haha).Looks like for the first time ever (EVER) I will wear a bikini on holiday (at least people will not see me again after the holiday!)Neil is not really into sun bathing on the beach (nor me as such) but I know the kids are looking forward to making some sandcastles. I cannot wait!!!!!!

Thursday 24th July 2003

Am counting the days. Am just managing to not stuff my face each day in stress (the kids have only been home since Tuesday after school)....I keep finding myself mysteriously in the kitchen just about to eat something (anything). Did a 2 hour line dance class last night so have at least had some exercise. Went shopping yesterday and looked at some swimwear, but think I have enough already. The temp is going to be in the 70's apparently (partly cloudy) am hoping the sun comes out a lot and can really feel like we are abroad!(ok we are but I do know it is possible to have 2 weeks of rain over there!).

Friday 25th July 2003

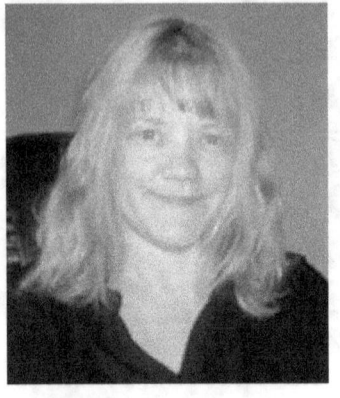

Worked in the shop today, Nicky gave me a chocolate roll, so that is my sins for the day. Have been on a 'green' day and have done well so far, 'cept Neil has just gone and got fish and chips for him and the kids and they smell lovely.. They are so hard to resist and I know I will probably eat a few (Just a few...honest!)

Sunday 27th July 2003

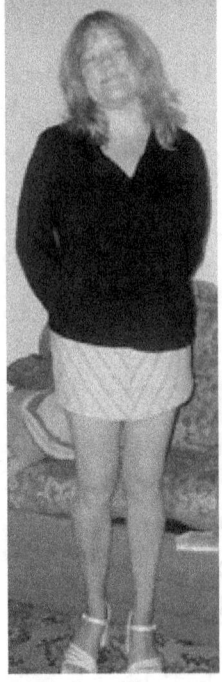

Here I am showing off my new sandals for the holiday! And here is Neil eating those chips I mentioned (I ate just 3 of them!!) But the kids went to my mums and slept there last night so Neil and I had Chinese and watched a new Clint Eastwood film Bloodwork and shared a few crisps too.

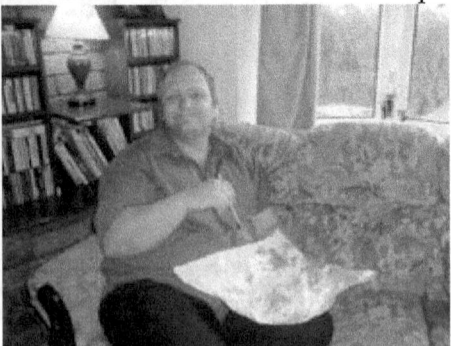

Slimming World Week 91

Monday 27th July 2003

I am hoping to have lost a lb this week (fingers crossed!)I have tried to be good but not always managed. I do not think I have lost more than a lb, I will be happy with a lb.

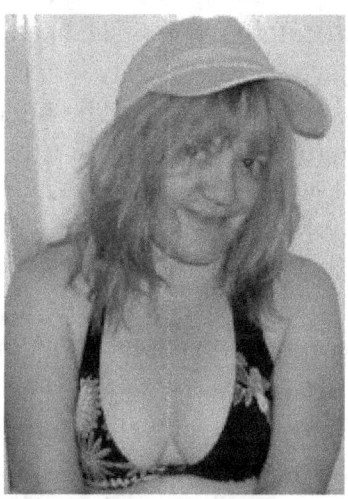

Here I am, I have the bikini's, the naff pink hat and am not totally white (so have a bit of a head start)...now all I need is a nice holiday in France!

Slimming World Weigh-In
Weight= 8 st 5 lbs (117 lbs)
Loss= 5 lbs
Still to lose= 5 lbs+

Monday evening - OK, my body is officially weird, truly it is. I have lost 5 lbs, I got weighed this morning and had lost 5 lbs.....just like that. HOW? Perhaps for all the times I was not so good, I was VERY good? I did eat a lot of fruit last week, especially grapes and strawberries. But 5 lbs.?

Went swimming today, not that I swam much as was looking after R, but it was nice to go to the pool(have not been for ages). Had a yummy options drink afterwards (chocolate and low fat), nice and hot and sweet and just 2 and a half sins. I really did not expect to have lost 5 lbs this week and it did cross my mind this morning...thoughts like (oh am I ill? Do I have a disease I do not know about?) When you have had sooooo many years of being overweight (without trying too hard!) it can be difficult to see yourself slimmer and keeping it off (without trying too hard).

Am totally looking forward to the holiday, have packed mainly for the sun (ok, almost totally for the sun, and I expect I should pack ONE waterproof thingy.....

Am tempted to treat myself with JUST a teeny weeny cream cake tonight...but shall try to resist (as Neil has gone to shop to get some, in case I just HAVE to have one...you know how it is, and it's just that time of the month too)

Will I resist?

Well, I could go on the railwalker tonight for my 'sins'! It is out from behind the couch (was showing it to my friend Nicola) and my knees are ok, so perhaps if I do give in to a bit of cake I will go on the railwalker... ok!

Ok, OK I admit it, I had 1 chocolate éclair (cake), and a bit of another cream cake (not much, it was not that nice). It's funny really just how much of a thing you can have when you don't really like it isn't it

Well, not long till my 40th birthday (18th August) at least I won't be FAT and FORTY! The holiday comes before my 40th so have not thought about becoming 40 as yet! EEEEKKKKK

Wednesday 30th July 2003

I am stressed already. The kids have been up 10 minutes and are fighting and I am argggggggghhhhhhhh. I have my 2 hr linedancing class tonight (this will help me chill out)...but have got the whole day to get through, even the thought of our up and coming holiday does little to reduce my stress levels at the moment. Luckily (or un luckily) we have very little in the cupboards (i.e. food) so I cannot go to the kitchen in frustration (stress). Although it is only 10am, if we had had stuff in, I think by now I would have been downstairs in a flash eating in anger. When the kids (R who is almost 6 and J who is 12) fight that is what is inclined to make me 'stress eat'. And all they seem to do lately is squabble constantly.

What is it with me at the moment? I am so narky...so angry (ah could be having the kids home and they are getting on my nerves)? I feel so ready to explode. I have eaten 2 white bread (which I normally avoid), some nougat and a chocolate biscuit - this has been my days eating, not good.

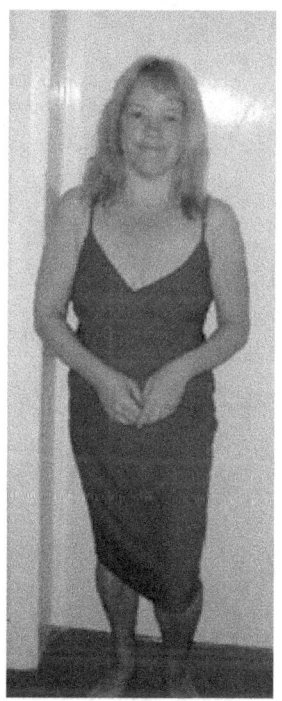

Bought this red dress from EBay and it came today and fitted nicely I am pleased to say (but am wearing holderinnerknickers....shushhhhhh!)

Thursday 31st July 2003

Eating pattern, what eating pattern? I do think I will probably eat better ob holiday than I am doing at the moment. Neil said to me last night after he got home "I have bought a surprise for you". Awwww nice...well, no not really, he had bought me a big bag of malteasers (chocolate), why? Arggghghghg. I did eat some of them, but gave most of them to J and his friend and R. Went linedancing last night and it was good, if tiring.

Sunday 3rd August - Sunday 17th August 2003

Hi Everyone, well this 2 weeks I am on holiday (Benodet, France) and hopefully I am chilling out and showing off the bits of my body I am ok with. And swimming in the pools, lazing on the beaches, doing lots of walking. Eating as healthily as I can (all that fresh fruit and vegetables and salad.) And hopefully we are all having fun and relaxing at the same time. There are a few pools on site, a tennis court, an adults only jacuzzi, you can hire bikes....there's some lovely beaches and walks to do. I hope the weather is good...but we are determined to make the most of it no matter what. See you all when I get back (am getting weighed on Monday 18th August which incidentally is also my 40th Birthday).

Slimming World Week 93

Monday 18th August 2003

MY 40th BIRTHDAY!

Well, here I am back from my holiday (how much have I gained?) And today I am 40.

We had a great time on holiday (can't stop singing the Chihuahua song by DJ Bobo) which is No 1 over most of Europe (not UK though).

> Slimming World Weigh-In
> Weight= 8 st 5 lbs
> STAYED THE SAME!
> Lbs to lose= would like to lose about 9 more

Well I have just come back from getting weighed and am pleased to say I stayed the same (yes after 2 weeks in France)! Neil is in work, we are skint (i.e. no money), he won't be back till late (probably) and I don't wanna be 40 (but am NOW). Ah well. Shall I go on? Make it a big moan? OK. Family are all on hol....as I said, no money, bugger all food in house (well perhaps that is a good start to me getting back to dieting!). My mum has forgotten to send me a card (she said "no one really celebrates birthdays when you get to this age"). Ermmmmm.....parents-in-law got me a card with a flower on it and said they didn't think I would want a 40th birthday one. OK moan over. I shall just sit here all day and aim to stop the kids from squabbling and try not to feel sorry for myself.

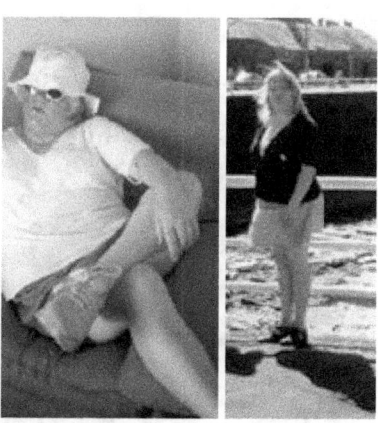

Gosh here I am on holiday 2001 in Devon so glad I didn't look like that this year!!

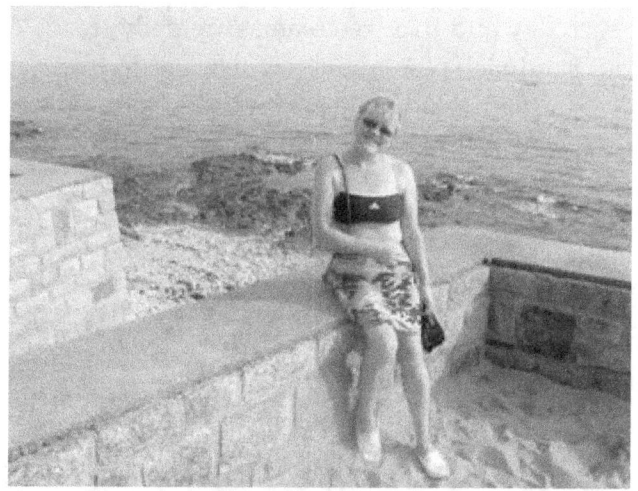

Here I am on Benodet beach just down from the site Camp St Gilles. We had fantastic weather for the whole 2 weeks.

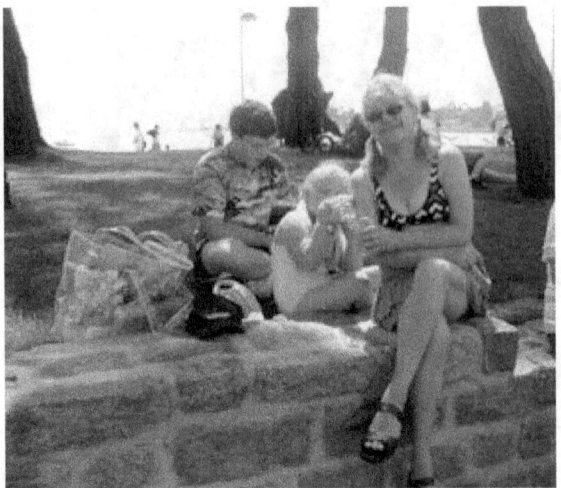

This was taken down in Benodet itself. We walked here almost each day and had ice-creams (my daily treat!) And we ate from a sandwich place (ham baguettes of course!)

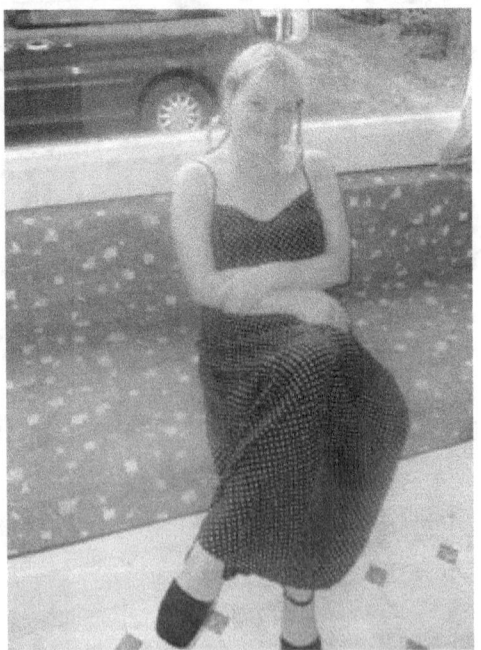

Here I am sitting in the caravan, we were just about to go out to the camp Club for the night. This is the night Neil actually got up and danced. He even did the Village People song YMCA!!!

Tuesday 19th August 2003

Everyone more or less ignored my 40th birthday. Neil never got home till after midnight. I felt very down, it was not how I imagined my BIG birthday to be... ah well, it is over now and gone so better forgotten. Now today I have to get back to following the SW plan, which is difficult after not following it for over 2 weeks. I start my college course on Sept 8th so I think it will be easier to follow the plan then (no picking at home!!!). So I may move my target to 7 lbs lower, don't know yet.

A funny day all in all. Did very little but lay around feeling sorry for myself again. Have had my 2 B choices (all for brekky)..had some salad and meat for lunch, that's about it. It is now almost 10pm.

Wednesday 20th August 2003

Had my toast for brekky (exciting eh!)

Am feeling soooooo down, totally totally down, bloody hell.

Had a good day yesterday, as I stuck to the plan. Did so much walking on hol and have now come to a dead stop....might get on the railwalker today (if I can muster up the energy), but I do have Linedancing tonight (I think), though part of me can't be bothered (arghghghghghghghhghhgh)

Don't think I will go to class (dancing) tonight, simply not in the mood. Did a small shop off Tesco and am pleased to say am avoiding all I bought - i.e. the breads/donuts/biscuits and such. Having no appetite helps.

Feeling brighter (now at 11pm) Have been chatting to Neil about how I feel (got it all off my chest so to speak). We watched a good film with Arthur Askey (one of my faves, Neil got it for me) And feel loads better. My friend Kim phoned and asked me to go round for coffee tomorrow too and Neil and I are booked to go see the new film Pirates of the Caribbean on Friday night and have just read Siobhan's nice entry into my guestbook.

Thank you to Siobhan for her kind words. That was really nice of you. I do feel better actually (amazing what a good film and a few nibbles can do!)

I was silly to let things get to me...I realise now.

Friday 22nd August 2003

Had a chocolate bikkie attack yesterday (mega) so do not expect to lose weight this Monday (that combined with cinema tonight and a meal out tomorrow night - all in aid of late birthday celebrating). I can make good choices at the meal and perhaps limit myself to sharing a popcorn at the pictures, so damage will be limited, but as I said, lack of exercise and 'picking' may result in a gain this coming week. Got the holiday pics back yesterday and it is nice to look at them an not cringe at myself (how I look), in most of them I look ok!!! Am at the shop this morning (for the last time).

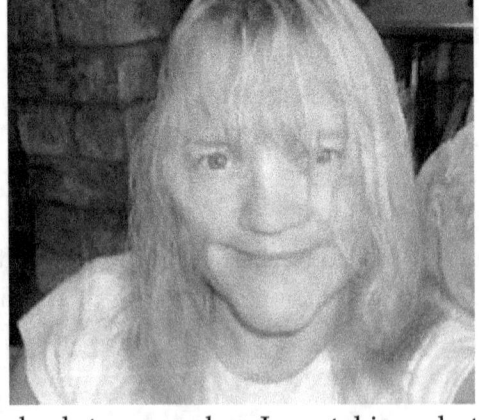

Must be back to normal as I am taking photos of myself again!!!!!!!! Haha!!! Here I am before going out to the cinema. Had a good day in the shop and the Boss Dave went out and got flowers for me from them all (belated bday), which was nice. Got a gorgeous long black 'officey' jacket for when I do my course which is a size 12 (US 8 to 10), fits lovely. Will share some popcorn with Neil tonight, we are going to see Pirates.

Slimming World Week 94

Monday 25th August 2003

Well, here we are again. I know for certain I have gained this week cos I ate SO much last week, with my birthday n all. We went out for a meal on the Saturday night, I was good but sampled a few cocktails and some wine and lager and then the cinema again on the Sunday (so nibbles).I am sure that when I get going to college every day my weight will settle down and I should (I say should) get to a weight I want to be and well....stay there. That's the plan!!

> Slimming World Weigh-In
> Weight = 8 st 7 lbs (119 lbs)
> Gain = 2 lb
> Lbs lost so far = 47 lbs
> (3 st 5 lbs)
> Lbs to lose = Want to lose about 7 to 10 more lbs

Not too bad, I gained just 2 lbs, I was convinced I had gained at least 4 lbs with all the eating I have done this last week. I am starting the eve class next week. Had some mince in the fridge so have made some yummy burgers (with all manor of herbs and onions etc), they are chilling in the fridge and are free on an Original day (am looking forward to these later!!

This is the last week I will be getting weighed in the morning (as I start college soon). I will move to Mon eve classes, so will still be getting weighed....but no longer doing the weighing (will miss this).

Tuesday 26th August 2003

Joined another MSN group, a Slimming World one, called Jo and Sue's Slimming World Class Flint (hey, my old home town). I love SW site's, the MSN groups, they are so helpful and there is always someone there to help when you most need it, all the people are in the same boat (i.e. trying to lose weight/maintain weight etc). In times when I have struggled I have come up here and sat at my computer and written (posted) to the groups....it has always helped. They are there for support/motivation and fun and friendship....most definitely worth joining.

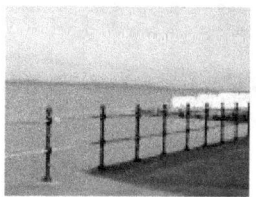

I am saying 'cheers' here, 'cept with a can of diet coke!!! One of our class consultants said Pepsi Max is a kind of diuretic (make you wee)....and it's sugar free therefore I have tins and tins of it in at any given time!!!!

Online friends HELP so much when you are trying to lose weight, they are invaluable

Thursday 28th Aug 2003

I said to myself the other day (night?) whenever, I said I will stick to the plan this week (haven't), I will spend less cash (haven't), I will test my blood sugars and do better with my insulin (ok, HAVE done some testing YEAHHHHH). But....have been out a fair bit and it is not always easy to eat how you mean to when you are out, but I do my best.

Here is West Kirby Marine Lake where I took the kids yesterday, had an ice-cream, sat on the beach flying a kite. Then had some lunch in a cafe (omelette and chips - ooops). But I did go linedancing last night for 2 hours!. Today I went to my friend's for lunch (we had pizza, something I rarely if ever have) and ok...chips, but not a huge amount. Need to get back on track!!!!!!!!!!

Sunday 31st August 2003

We went on a day trip yesterday. I took along butties, but when we came to eat them they were so soggy and yuck, I threw them away. So instead I ordered a pasta and salad dish at the cafe (rather fattening I am sure...but nice). I ate a jelly for dessert (so yum and cold)and had diet drinks. I did nibble throughout the day unfortunately (a polo mint here, a crisp there). But we walked a fair bit and had a really nice day out (me and the kids on a trip to Manchester Museum of Science and Industry)

Slimming World Week 95

Here we are into September

Monday September 1st 2003

I am getting weighed this evening (changing to eve class), therefore it is logical that I will automatically weigh more this week, as I always weigh about 2 lbs heavier in the evening. So, it is probable that I will have to pay this week, as I can only gain 3 lbs in this weigh in (no more)...if I have gained less than 3 lbs then I am still in the target so do not have to pay. But. given I have not stuck to the plan every day, I certainly feel I have gained more then 3 lbs. But I will not worry...I will get back on track. That is the difference now, I feel fine about any gains (ok, a bit disappointed), but in the past I would have gone and eaten (binged in frustration and hating myself for having gained)...now it is different. I know I can do it, I know I can eat well and still lose with the SW plan...so any weight gain NO PROBLEM!

Today I go to enrol in college for my 1 yrs Office Admin Course...I am sooo looking forward to this.

Slimming World Weigh-In
Weight = 8 st 8 lbs
Gain= 1 lb (I can live with this!)
Lbs lost so far – 146 lbs (3 st 4 lbs)
Lbs to lose = 10 ish

Enrolled at college. Then this evening I went to the SW class and got weighed...I only had a gain of 1 lb which is great. I am now going back on track and raring to go. Have a different consultant now. Angela.

Wednesday 3rd September 2003

Kids go back to school tomorrow!!!!!! I am trying to eat well, but we have not been shopping and there isn't a lot in, on the other hand that means there also isn't much of anything to tempt me either. When you are not organised with the eating you almost always end up eating stuff you didn't mean to, it is far far better to plan and have the stuff in.

I am hungry because I don't have the 'free foods' in

Thursday 4th September 2003

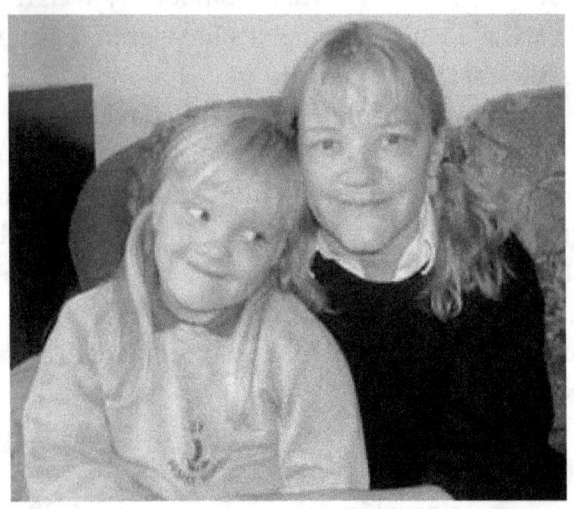

Here is R and I today, she enjoyed her 1st day back at school. So did J. I did some gardening tonight (exercise) although I did have 2 or was it 3 chocolate biscuits.

Saturday 6th September 2003

I am struggling to eat properly at the moment for a number of reasons, the main one being we are having money probs and just cannot go do a decent shop at the moment, so I am eating just what's left in the cupboards and why is it that 'fatty' foods, junk foods are so much cheaper than healthier stuff? I am trying but it is not easy. Also I have terrible toothache (have been to dentist) and I require a LOAD of treatment (hey estimated bill £372.00 and this is the NHS). I am taking antibiotics for a tooth infection and it hurts like hell to chew (so am trying to avoid chewing). Have eaten a lot of porridge lately, ok, not terribly fattening but is not a good choice on the Slimming World plan. I have my fave Muller yogs in but they set off the toothache (argghghghghghghgh).

Slimming World Week 96

How the weeks are flying by!

Monday 8th September 2003

I start my course today (this week is induction week). Am aiming to go and get weighed tonight but may not be able to make it??? Will do my best. I am looking forward to going to college (am taking butties tomorrow!).

Well I took the butties to college but the stuff in the canteen was sooooooooooooooo much nicer! I had a brown ham batch with coleslaw (I love coleslaw). It was great at college, I think this is going to be the best thing I have done for ages (besides going to Slimming World that is). There's about 20 or so of us on the course, varying ages. The course tutor Morag is really nice, she seems the sort to really want the best for us all and want us all to do well (of course we HAVE to out the effort in). I am looking forward to this year. I must admit I am still not sure if I am going to go tonight. I need a good week, a good weightloss and this won't be the week for it (my own fault).

I need to follow the plan properly, I meant to have done it this last week...I DID NOT and so feel a bit naffed off with myself.

> Slimming World Weigh-In
> Weight = 8 st 7 lbs
> Loss/Gain = 1 lb
> Lbs I want to lose still = About 10

Think I have been eating too much of the wrong things lately.

Wednesday 10th September 2003

As you can see I actually lost a lb this week (yesssss). I made myself go to the class and I also stayed (keeps me motivated!). Am in the middle of my induction week at college and really enjoying it and totally looking forward to well...learning again!

Am going to Linedancing tonight, my exercise.

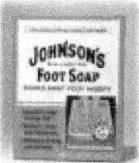

My feet survived the Linedancing class!

Saturday 13th September 2003

College went fine this week. If I eat in the canteen I try to make sure it is healthy (mainly I have a ham or chicken batch, minus the butter). The times I get tempted are, when I am on my way to the bus station, I often feel like getting just ONE small chocolate thing (anything!), but am trying to resist. I am still in the habit of picking and need to stop doing this if I want to lose any more weight. I feel quite flabby at the moment and seem to be trying to hide my tummy all the time.

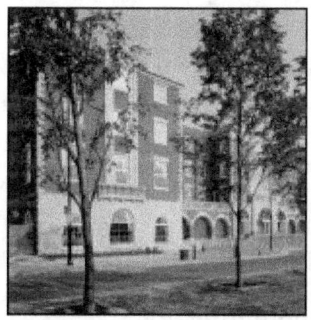

Here is the college that I go to. I have to bus it here each day, it is quite a pleasant college, relatively new.

Slimming World Week 97

I will eat healthier and cook better stuff

Monday 15th September 2003

Have the dentist to look forward to this week (boo hoo). I am just about to go and get weighed, I suspect I have gained some, but I am determined to get back on the plan. Had a ham sandwich in college today and asked for 'a little amount' of coleslaw but got LOADS, nice though!

Went and got weighed and stayed to the meeting, I am glad I went, I enjoyed it. This week we were asked what would we (did we) treat ourselves too when we lose (lost) our weight? I said I really want a 1940's makeover, that is what I want more than anything.

Slimming World Weigh-In
Weight = 8 st 5 lbs (117 lbs)
Loss= 2 lbs
Lbs I still want to lose= about 7 lbs

Yep, if I lose 7 lbs that will take me to 7 st 12 lbs (110 lbs). I want to be 7 st something. I know if I make the effort and stick to the plan then I can achieve this. Though weirdly I feel FATTER at the moment and EVEN look fatter (even Neil agreed with this - humphhhh!)

Arghghghghghhg have not done my CV for college yet!

Wednesday 17th September 2003

Neil came home with some chocolates from work, ok so I ate some, but have been doing my best to get the kids to eat them so I don't have to (aren't tempted!) I did some gardening yesterday (with a HUGE petrol mower) so - good exercise.

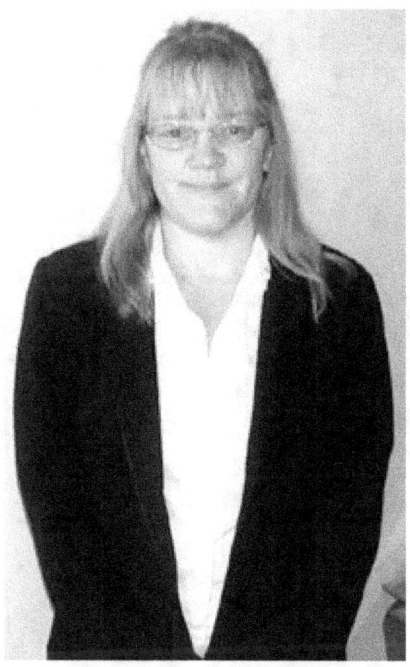

Here I am about to go to college this morning. We have to wear lavender blouses (I bought one today at the market - we all have to wear the same blouses), I shall have to do a pic of me in the proper blouse.

Saturday 20th September 2003

Went to Blackpool today with the Diabetes group, had a nice day out, though ate too much or rather the wrong things.

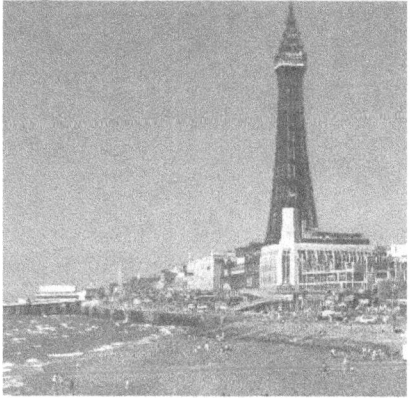

Here's Blackpool Tower, I went to the top (well almost the top!)

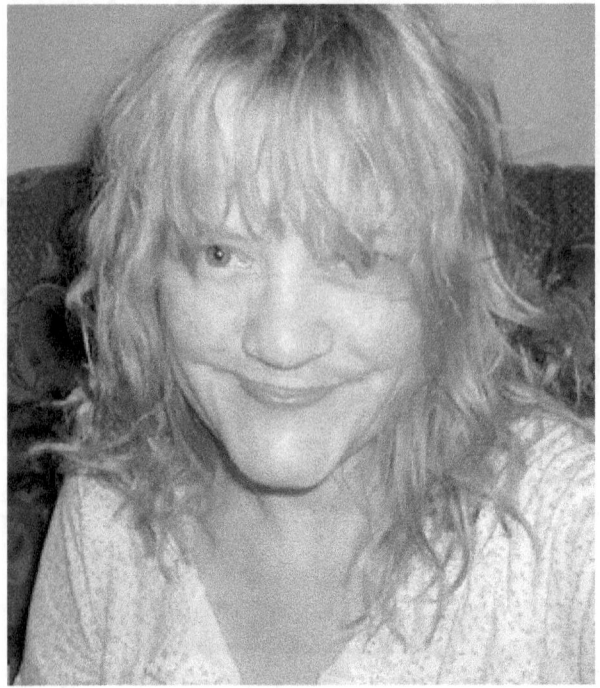

Me after my trip to Blackpool (tired)

I had chips (not too many), a pastie (have not had one of these for years), some more chips and shepherds pie with mushy peas, a stick of rock and a penguin biscuit....that is all, so perhaps not too bad????????

Slimming World Week 98

Monday 22nd September 2003

I am going to make a huge effort to be the weight I want to be for Christmas (or sooner). I am going to eat properly, none of this picking and I am going to get better control of my blood sugars. Sure, I am maintaining, but I do want to lose about 10 more lbs and I desperately need to test my blood sugars more (I eat far too many sweet things).

Saw Pirates of the Caribbean twice and would like to see it a third time (I am sad!).

> Slimming World Weigh-In
> Didn't go to get weighed this week, blame it on Neil!

Tuesday 23rd September 2003

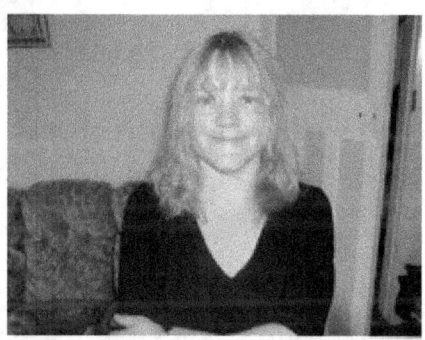

Went to college as usual... am feeling v tired! I took my lunch with me (ham butty) but after I had eaten it a friend came and sat by me eating sausage and mash with onion gravy (only £1.00) Oh I just had to have some...so I went and got some!

Today was ok...did lots of walking. Though I feel my college blouse is a tad too tight (arghghghgh).......I want to be 7st something NOW.

Thursday 25th September 2003

I have to go have a tooth out today and I promised myself I would not get worked up about it...but it is 8.30 in the morning and breakfast is not settling well in my stomach......am having the tooth out at 2.45pm. I am so dreading it (silly) and even worse I have to have 2 out together next week.

I will not get worked up... I will be calm.

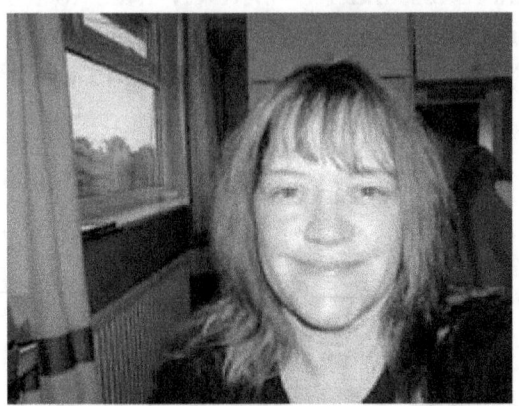

The hair saga continues!! Ok... gone a bit darker (the other day).

Decided to go for having the 2 teeth out at once, one came out fine, didn't even realise she'd done it... but the other... well, it is still in my mouth (half of it) it simply would not come out and after about 6 injections and lots of pulling and tugging she gave up, plus it was hurting me loads by then (despite enough novocaine to take all the teeth out). She said I have an infection so have to take a course of antibiotics and come back next week . So I go back to try again and have another one out also (3 altogether)..I feel icky.

Slimming World Week 99

It is Sunday night (Sunday 28th September 2003) and here I am having eaten badly all day despite my teeth hurting (I managed). I had made some leek and potato soup for a green day, slept in bed and Neil brought me up some lunch (ham sandwich - red day). The fridge had chocolate biscuits in it - I ate them, not all of them, felt too sick for that. Weighed myself on my scales and appear to have gained 4 or 5 lbs, jumped off the scales.

I am going to go and get weighed in the morning (no, not because you weigh lighter in the mornings, no)..but because I am going into college late cos I have a hospital appointment for my diabetic clinic. Ok so getting weighed in the morning will be less of a shock to me... I will still have gained of course.

Monday 29th September 2003

Ok, so what damage have I done? I will get back on track, I have to mainly cos my college blouse is getting too tight and I don't want to buy the next size.)

> Slimming World Weigh In
> Weight= 8 st 9 lbs (121 lbs)
> Gain= Yes I gained 4 lbs
> Lbs to lose = about 12

As you can see my bad eating has caught up with me and I gained 4 lbs. Not to worry, I will get it off again, I know I can do it. I am much more confident about my ability to lose weight and nowadays gaining weight (if I know the reason why) does not bother me half as much as it used to).

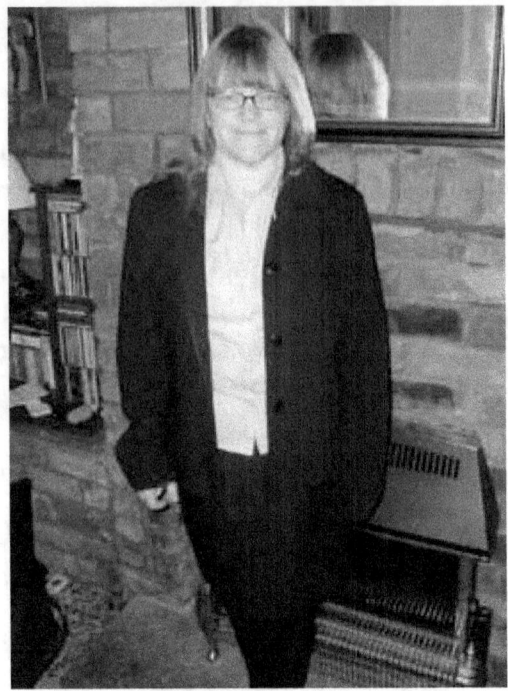

Me ready to go to college

Tuesday 30th September 2003

Toothache is so horrible. I have been taking painkillers every 4 hours and eating and drinking sets it off, this tooth that needs to come out (half tooth that they couldn't get out last Thursday). Trouble is I think another tooth is kicking in too and might need to come out, or perhaps it is what they call referred pain? I think I can hold out till next Thursday? If the tooth does not come out easily they will refer me to the hospital (I would rather go there first so they do not have to try to get it out at the dentist). I have eaten very little today, Neil came home from work early and I went to bed. I am back in college tomorrow (hopefully will help to take my mind off the teeth problem)..so armed with co-codomol I should be ok.

When I am asleep it is easier to diet!!!!!!!!!!!!!!!

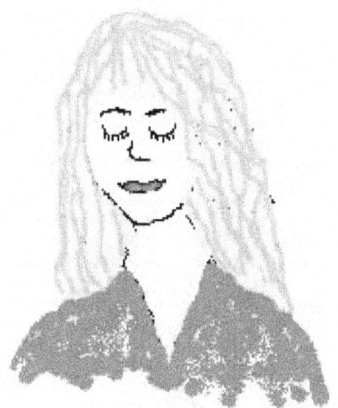

I have started doing my own little cartoons (above) and am going to do loads of them and put them on the site and all on a separate page for people to use if they want.

Thursday 2nd October 2003

College was ok today. I have managed to stick to the plan so far, but am craving anything chocolate and there is nothing similar in the house (arghghghghghg).

The Coffee Diet

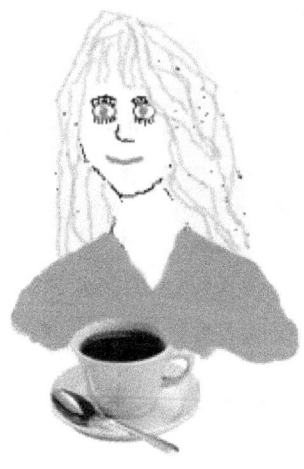

See here is another one of my little cartoons, I cannot think of a name for the character (so suggestions welcomed!)

Friday 3rd October 2003

Had a breakfast in college, didn't mean to, but I did. I do admit to having a chocolate attack last night, I ate loads and yes my blood sugars were high as a result. I just ate far too much of it. I cannot turn back the clock (no fair).

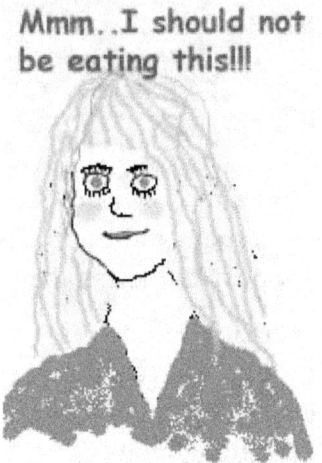

I have decided to do a new site...much like this one really. I have decided I need to redo this site so am in the middle of setting up a new one, I did not want to just change this one....so when the new one is ready this one will no longer be available. As I said the new one is very much the same. I felt this one was getting too big and I don't suppose many (if any) people go back to the beginning of my weeks to see them).

Slimming World Week 100

Monday 6 October 2003

Here we are again, almost time (in an hour) for another weigh-in. I realise I have not been so good on my diet this past week.....I started the week off well but lost the plot half way through, so I guess I will certainly have another gain. I am still in the process of doing the new web site, but I hope to have it done by the end of this week, so then this one will no longer be available.

> Slimming World Weigh-In
> Weight this week= 8 st 6 lbs (118 lbs)
> Loss= YES! 3 lbs
> Lbs I want to lose= about 10 lbs

I am happy now!

Can you believe it, I actually lost 3 lbs. Maybe I wasn't as bad as I thought! Ok I came home and had a small (just a small) portion of chips (say 1/4 of a bag) and 1/2 a fish. Oh and I did buy a pack or two of the Slimming World new Mince Pie Hi Fi Bars (and ok I ate 4 of them - they are yummy). So not counting the chips the bars are 22 sins or 4 B choices (oooops). That's it, pig-out over, the rest of the wee I am going to eat sensibly for once, for once (in a long time) I am actually going to count sins. I have been following the Red/Green day basics but not paying too much attention to those 'sins'. At college today I had a chicken batch (brown - no spread) and a bowl of mixed salad (ok it had a tablespoon of coleslaw in it)!

Saturday 11th October 2003

Had my difficult tooth out (yippeee) Have been eating FAR too MUCH chocolate for my liking (well, I do like actually)....but too much. Also last night I had some Baileys mini drinks (yummy), had ermmmm 4 of these (oh how I hate to admit it to myself!). I will, I will have a good week, I will - I need a good week cos this snacking and picking and eating the wrong things is sneaking back in too often.

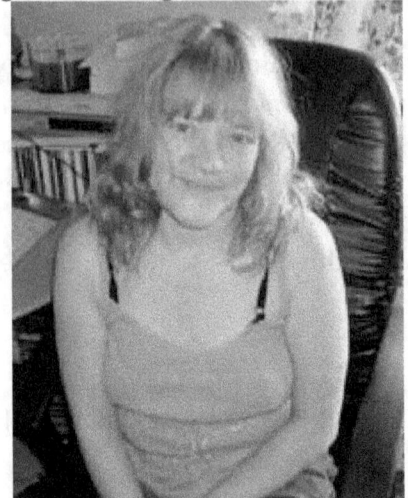

Can you tell I have no teeth in here!
Honestly I don't (he he).

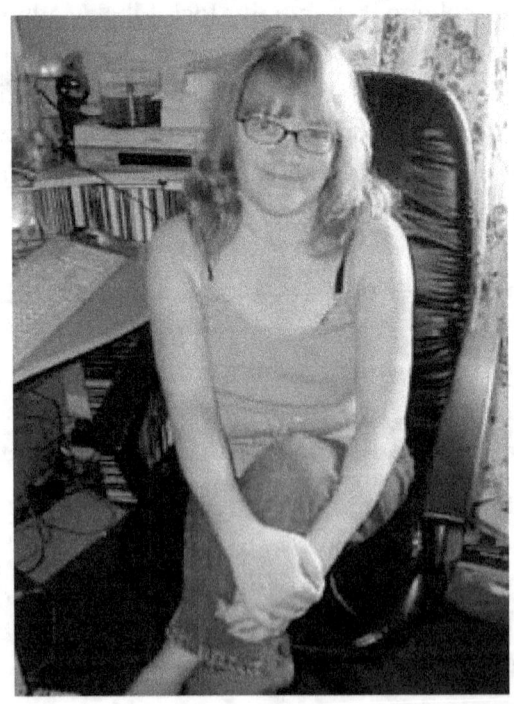

I actually got up at 7.30 this morning and was painting the kitchen (as you do). Well it's all exercise isn't it.

Editor's Note.
Cathy's old website finishes at this point and everything moves to the new website. The dates continue unbroken.

Monday 13th October to Sunday 19th October

Sunday 12th October 2003

It was R's 6th birthday part today, we had a Harry Potter themed one and we did experiments, two of the mums stayed to help me (thank goodness)! It all went well.

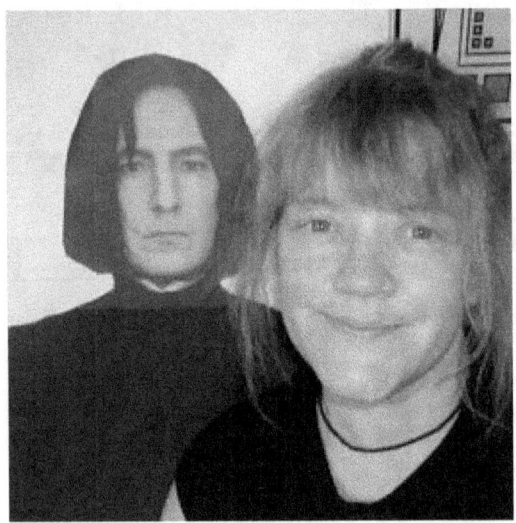

Some photos taken today (Sunday). I hung candles from the ceiling with invisible thread (very spooky!) - the kids liked it.

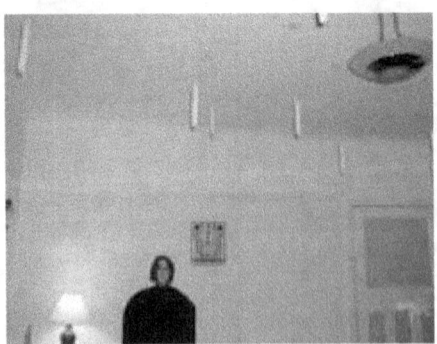

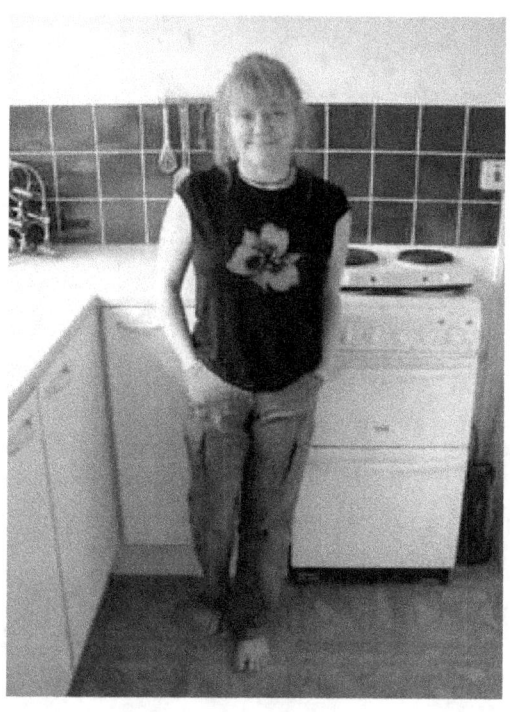

It is just gone half past 8 in the evening (I am knackered!)

Monday 13th October 2003

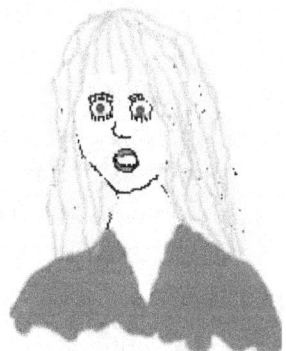

Weight this week is 8 st 7 lbs (119 lbs)
I have lost 47 lbs since November 2001
I want to lose about 10 more lbs

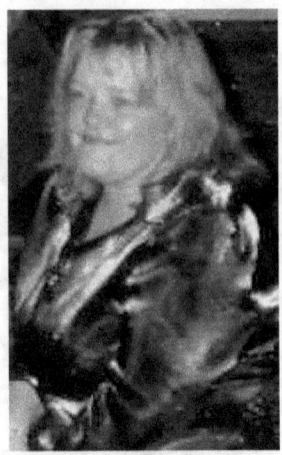

Me when I started Slimming World back in November 2001. I weighed about 11 st 4 lbs here (158 lbs), this was taken at a Christmas party.

If I am honest, I do not want to go and get weighed tonight because of all the chocolate eating I have been doing. But I will go and I will get weighed and I will do better this coming week.

Ok, just a lb and I am glad I went to the meeting, I feel more motivated now. We are having a 'taster' session next week so I am going to make my fave recipe - corned beef bol (minus the spaghetti).

Tuesday 14th October 2003

Funny day really, went to college, felt a bit stressed and came home feeling 'totally' down in the dumps, but have managed to keep away from the kitchen!

I have a meeting tonight, another tomorrow night and one the night after!! PHEW. All connected with the diabetic group. Oh and another tooth out on Thursday (and a kid to tea Thursday night)and and and............

Wednesday 15th October 2003

Went to my diabetic meeting tonight, we had a talk on the heart/hypertension, it was very interesting. College was fine today, I missed lunch but had it when I got home at 2.30 pm. In my diabetic meeting I was craving choccy (what's new?)

and had a snickers bar.......was it worth it? No not really, I ate it so quickly I hardly had time to taste it. Sometimes I should think twice before giving in to a whim of wanting chocolate. Well on the plus side I was going to get a few bars of chocolate besides the snickers bar and I didn't - so that is good NO? YES!

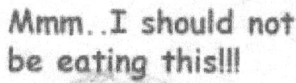

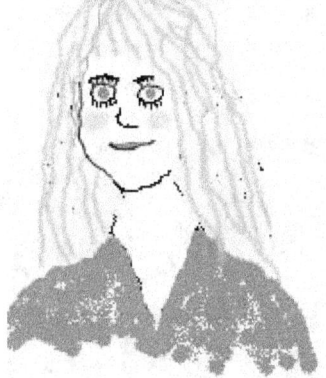

I need to stock up on healthy snacks in the fridge and cupboards, then I am less likely to eat silly things that make me gain weight.

Friday 17th October 2003

Had my hair cut today, on the spur of the moment. Sometimes it is nice to have a change, now tomorrow I will want longer hair!!!!! Did well eating till on the way home then bought myself 2 choccy things. Last night I had a meeting and over did the biscuits....where is my self control????

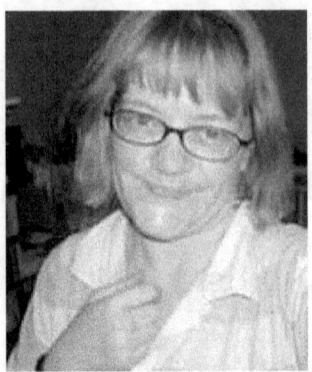

Oh I do wish I could stop 'snacking'...I am doing it far too often.

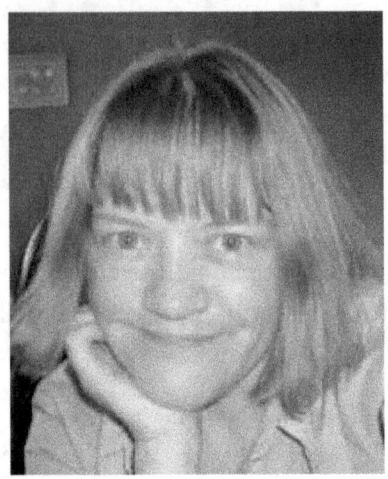

Saturday 18th October 2003

Arhghghghghghgh, I have the decent food in, I cannot eat properly...no reason not to, it's just my brain cannot get into gear!! Ok, Ok, tomorrow (yes tomorrow tomorrow) I will eat properly. I sort of want to eat just whatever I want without thinking about it (ever) and well, this is sort of what I am doing, but I wish I could do this but eat the right things not junk food and chocolate etc. Eat what I want when I want - all healthy stuff, ermmmm like salad and veggies and stuff????? The sort of food that does not make you gain weight. But unfortunately this is not the sort you want to eat late at night watching television is it?!

Sunday 19th October 2003

Went to my mum and dads today, had a few sweeties (but managed to NOT eat a chocolate biscuit in my sisters, ah just remembered....had 3 jaffa cakes in my mums (bugger). She made me a chicken salad for lunch, that was healthy.

Week 2

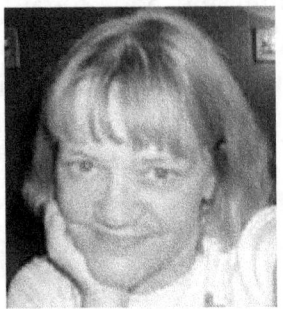

Ok, not week 2 exactly. I mean, I have been going to Slimming World for almost 2 years now and have lost 47 lbs in this time, going from

11 st 12 lbs to 8 st 7 lbs. I am aiming to keep going to SW each week and I would really like to lose another 10 lbs.

Monday 20th October 2003

Ok, once again, I just know I have gained weight, and I am fed up of saying this. I am fed up of not quite doing it right, not quite making the effort.

> Weight this week = 8 st 5 lbs (117 lbs)
> Loss= 2 lbs
> Lbs lost so far= 49 lbs
> Lbs to lose still= 7 to 10

Huh? Huh? I think my body is great, it has lost 2 lbs this week, despite me thinking it had gained weight. As Neil said, maybe just maybe I am not as bad as I think (eating wise). Maybe just maybe I make better choices than I realise? Looks like it doesn't it? Actually maintaining is not as hard as I thought it would be. I have been at target now for just over 5 months.

Am wondering what to wear for Halloween.

We are invited to a Halloween party at the Scout hut, along with my friend Judith and her 2 boys, she is arranging it. I do enjoy dressing up (any excuse!) and have been looking on EBay for a good outfit.

Friday 24th October 2003

Have been experimenting with looks for Halloween. We are going to McDonalds on the Friday night (31st) they have a Halloween party and on the Saturday night Judith (friend) her scout group is having a Halloween party too. FUN!

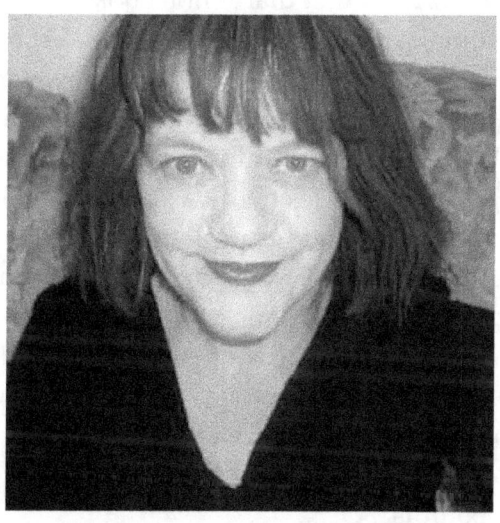

I have been trying my best to stick to the plan this week but not managing very well. I started a little notebook for Neil and I to write down what we are eating (plus our weight each week) - I filled in Mondays and that was it (eekkkkk). If I am to get to my new target of 7 st 12 lbs for Christmas, I need to stick to the SW plan properly, I know I can do it, it's just doing it!

Week 3 Halloween

Slimming World Weigh In
Weight= 8 st 7 lbs (119 lbs)
Gain= 2 lbs
Lbs lost so far= 47 lbs
Lbs to lose= 7 to 10

Monday 27th October 2003

Am getting weighed tonight and feel I have gained weight this week (yes again). My stomach is so bloated and feels yuck. We have all been sick actually (puking up bug). Today I have started a diet diary (notebook) to make a note of what I am eating, perhaps this will help me keep on track? As you can see I went and got weighed (did the weighing, which I really enjoyed) and yes I gained 2 lbs which I was not surprised about and don't mind too much as I know it will be gone next week (I hope)! Feel yuck as ate ermmm, what was it now? Oh yeah, some (lots) chocolate, a bit of (loads) mince and spaghetti (at least this was healthy)..also had some (4) Muller yoghurts (lemon n lime ones at least these are free). Bought some low fat custard (of non popular make i.e. not ambrosia or however you spell it) and was going to eat the whole tin (cold - yummy) but well, you know, it didn't taste quite nice so I was GOOD and didn't eat it, might have had a few large spoonfuls. SO......

Tomorrow....will be making notes in my little diet book (NOTE - must go buy a new funky little notebook to write what I am eating in when I go to Liverpool with friends tomorrow)

Tonight I am doing the weighing-in at the class (filling in cos the usual girl is not in)

At least I am not hungry now (this said at 8.30 pm at night after what I have eaten today)!

Thursday 30th October 2003

Here is a photo of me and the kids and my friend and her daughter when we went to Liverpool, we went to the museum and shopping! Yesterday I went to Southport and had lunch out (lasagne - very fattening). I have eaten out a lot this week and not always made good choices, I can feel it round my middle already. Funnily enough though, when I was out yesterday and Neil and I were going around Tesco at the end of the day, Neil accused me of being a stick! Me a stick.................ha. And someone Neil knows (i.e. Steve) said was I taking the dieting too far, that I looked gaunt. I DON'T THINK SO. I cannot win can I. Body image............my reflection tells me I am still a bit fat and need to lose more. Of course what's left is my tummy, all the fat left is round my middle and that is what I see, what I focus on and do not like. It makes me feel fat (and uncomfortable).

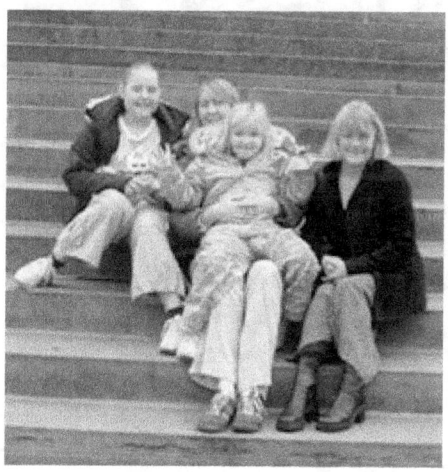

Having a day out

Sunday 2nd November 2003

Ate far too much yesterday, loads of stuff I would not normally eat (ah well) So I really really have to get sticking to the plan now. I tried on a dress I was going to wear for the Halloween party but it had gotten tight (OH NO). We went to a Halloween party last night then on to a family party where I had way too many nibbles.

Today I am going to eat properly (it's hard to get back into the habit when you have eaten just about whatever you want for a week (think it was a week). I KNOW I will have a weight gain tomorrow, I just know it and I hope it is no mote than 3 lbs (or I have to pay in my slimming club!). 3 lbs would take me to the top limit of my target. We shall see.

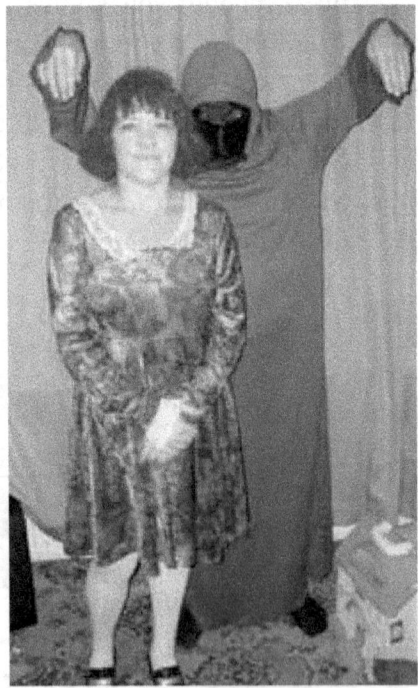

Me and J last night

Week 4 - Monday 3rd November to Sunday 9th November 2003

Monday 3rd November 2003

Was already NOT to go and get weighed when my conscience got the better of me and now I AM going. I know I have gained, hence putting gain on the right (even before I have gotten weighed). I am going to get weighed in about 20 minutes (Arhghghghghghg)

> Weight this week = 8 st 9 lbs (121 lbs)
> Gain = 2 lbs
> Lbs I want to lose = at least 12

As you can see I gained 2 lbs, that is what you get for too much snacking and a bottle of wine and oh a bottle of Bacardi Breezer (small one) and yeah, nibbles. So...............have started writing down what I am eating in a cute Barbie notebook (borrowed from R). I would like a loss next week. I collected the money at today's meeting, I am glad I went (had to force myself to go). Neil is also writing down what he is eating (ok I am doing it for him), when he wants to diet, I have to do most of the work for him, all but put the food in his mouth!

Tuesday 4th November 2003

Off to a meeting tonight......lots of cups of coffee!!! Called in out local newspapers office today to see about a work placement there in February, I have to send them a covering letter and CV (fingers crossed. Have managed to avoid chocolate today (was tempted but too lazy really to go from bus stop to shop (just wanted to get home!)

Thursday 6th November 2003

Had a nice email from Cerilyn in TX (USA) who says she has lost 66 lbs so far (WOW, well done) and she wished me good luck for keeping off the chocolate!!! Encouragement and support is greatly appreciated, even though I am at my target weight, I still need some help staying there. After all, I was overweight for over 12 years and certainly old habits can sneak back in and those little pounds can scarily pile back on if you are not careful. I do not have the metabolism to be able to eat what I want when I want (not counting having diabetes). Though I must say I never had a weight problem when I was younger then again this is common, many people say this. I really gained all my weight during my pregnancies. It is SO easy to gain a lb and another and another and before you know it, loads of them. Not fair is it, especially when it can seem so hard, impossible almost to get rid of lbs. You seem to have to work so very hard to lose a lb but can gain one when you don't even know how??

Some weeks I think Mmmmmmm I ate lots of 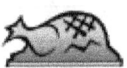 and lots of 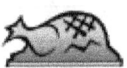 good sources of protein and I lose more weight when I eat more protein (am not talking about the Atkins diet here, just eating more lean meats) And I have more and other fruit and I certainly eat TONS of and generally on these sort of weeks, I do lose weight even if I have sneaked in the odd or like last night I had a

(OK I admit it, I had ermmmm 2). I have to satisfy my . Other weeks my eating is all over the place and I have very few veggies/fruit, I seem to snack a lot and pick a lot and eat WAY too much and these are the weeks I gain weight. I can put on weight and I seem to have cracked the losing of it and now I have to manage the keeping it off.

IT'S
EASY   isn't it???????

Saturday 8th November 2003

I have created a new page for the site, it is a sort of motivation form, a set of statements and things to do that may help people, well, I hope it might. If you do make use of the form do email me and tell me what you thought of it. THANKS!

Week 5

Monday 10th November to Sunday 16th November 2003

Monday 10th November 2003

Yes, here we are again, another weighing in day. I will say the usual and say I have gained weight, not good, not good at all. I am still hoping to have lost another 10 lbs plus by Christmas, I had better get a move on then hadn't I?

I am working in the office at college this week, I hope it will be a good week, I am looking forward to it. I actually wrote to a local newspaper hoping to get a placement there in February (as part of the college course I have to find myself a placement for 6-7 weeks work experience.) Perhaps because Neil works for a newspaper in Southport, is why the possibility of working in one interests me so? Neil doesn't actually do writing for the paper, he is one of their computer consultants and funnily enough Neil's work colleague used to work for the paper I am hoping to get a placement at - small world. Ah back to dieting....

Can I apply this to dieting? Certainly the more I say I will stick to it, the less I do. Perhaps I should fill in my own motivation sheet and put it on MY fridge!

How have I done this week? I had a good start to the week, really I did. But it went off somehow and towards the end of the week, well, I totally lost the good eating plan didn't I.

> Weight this week = 8 st 7 lbs
> Loss = 2 lbs
> Lbs I want to lose = about 10

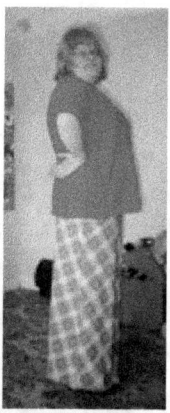

Year 2000 weighing about 11 st 12 lbs)
(166 lbs)

Wednesday 12th November 2003

Ah, see I was wrong, I actually lost 2 lbs this week. I am sure there are people out there wondering just what it is I have to moan about (with my weight)! I am rather pleased that I have managed to maintain my weightloss since May. It is difficult to like your body and feel ok with it sometimes, especially when you have been overweight for so long. I have well and truly learned to 'hate' the way I look. When I see myself in a mirror or shop window all I see is my stomach (the part I am unhappy with), I do not even glance at the rest of me, I see a HUGE stomach and that is what I think people see. When people (ok men.....let's be honest and yes I know I'm married) look at me (in passing) I believe they see a 'fat' person, because my tummy takes over, it is big and there and focusable on (maybe not a real word!?). My legs are skinny, my arms are ok, hair (well........) and face (double well.........???) but my tummy spoils everything, bummer or what! (ermmm...bum is ok size)

Moan over (for now)!!!!!!

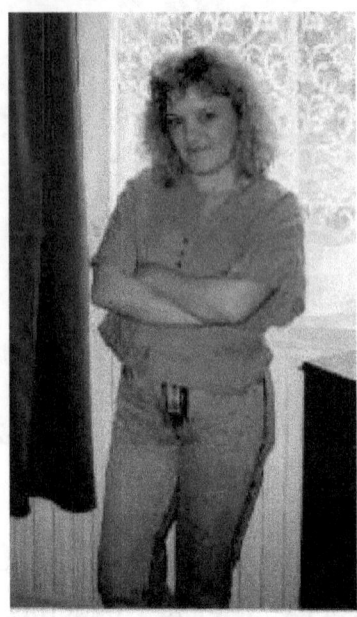

Here I am in 1990 when I met Neil, I weighed about 8 st
(112 lbs)

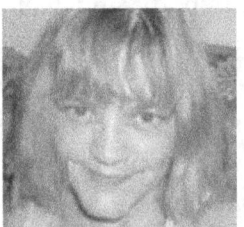

Here I am the other day weighing 8 st 7 lbs
(119 lbs)

Friday 14th November 2003

Have finished my first whole week in the Admin Bureau at college, I did enjoy it. Wore a longline jacket to college, thought I looked ok in it (and wore higher shoes so looked taller). Have not been to Linedancing for a few weeks and unfortunately cannot go this coming week as I have a diabetic meeting, I miss my exercise, plus it's enjoyable.

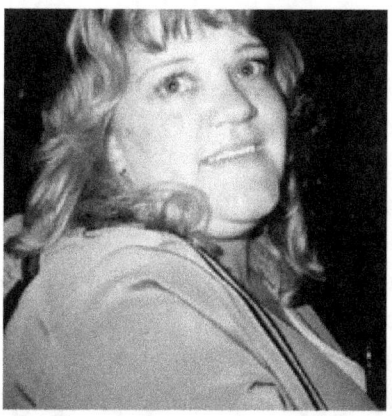

1995-ish at my sister's hen night I weighed about 12st
(168 lbs)

Monday 17th November through to Sunday 23rd November 2003

Monday (again) 17th November 2003

These Mondays seem to come around so quickly! I am in the middle of creating a 'diet game' and will be putting this on the site for people to print out.

Weight today =8 st 7 lbs (119 lbs)
Stayed the same
Lbs I STILL want to lose by Christmas = 10

Tuesday 18th November 2003

Am pleased to say I stayed the same weight this week (PHEW!) Now I am going to try (really try) and stick to the plan for the week, I have my dad's 60th birthday meal soon and want to lose some lbs so I can put some on, if you see what I mean! I have put up the game I created, ok so it is a 'snakes and ladders' type game so may get boring after a few games. I took it along to my SW class and the consultant Angela seemed impressed and I am doing some copies for her (she is going to laminate them). R (who is 6 wants to play the game tonight). A slimming one is not quite for her so I shall have to think of a suitable one for her, they are quite fun to make and will last for ages when laminated, you can certainly let your imagination run away with you (plus I love searching for suitable graphics).

I finished my week in the Admin Bureau, I did enjoy it, now it's back to work in the classroom.

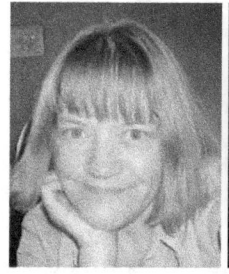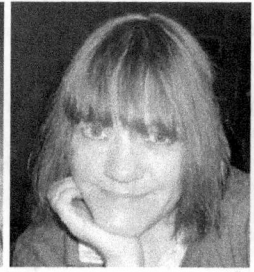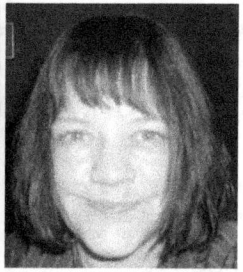

You may remember the hair saga from the other site? Well, we're off again.........! The latest colour is....ermm, the one on the far right. For the time being! Does it make my face look slimmer I wonder?

I am sure Neil must despair of me constantly taking pics of myself!! Ha ha and the constant hair colour changing, same as the house really.......I am always changing the colour of the rooms and Neil often comes home to, well, first the kitchen was yellow, then duck egg blue now white, all in quite a short space of time. Psychologically it may mean something?? Mmmmm. I wonder?

Thursday 20th November 2003

Arghghgh toothache again. Off to dentist today. After nibbling my way through at least (from what I can recall) 3 (small ok) chocolate bars yesterday, ones I had never bought before so had to do a taster of them.....I have decided enough's enough. No more choccy binges. I have to keep an eye on my blood sugars (certainly) and if I want to lose this last 10 lbs, well, NO chocolate except for the odd bit here and there. I am not eating fatty foods or lots of takeaways or that sort of thing, I am spoiling it by nibbles. Had almost a whole tube of Pringles (oh the awfulness of it) and best thing is I am not really a crisp (potato chip) fan. I have to make an effort instead of this dilly dallying.

Oops had chips tonight (well, as a treat cos I had been to the dentist, that's my excuse anyway!)

Friday 21st November 2003

Ok, ok had a Chinese takeaway tonight no rice... yes like that's good?), it is actually, I am on a red day...so there! Feel yuck now, I have eaten too much. Oh damn I had a snickers bar and ermm a small fruit and nut bar....now why did I have to remember those? So I guess I was not so good today (ooopppsss again). Hey, perhaps I will do some exercise tomorrow? What exercise?

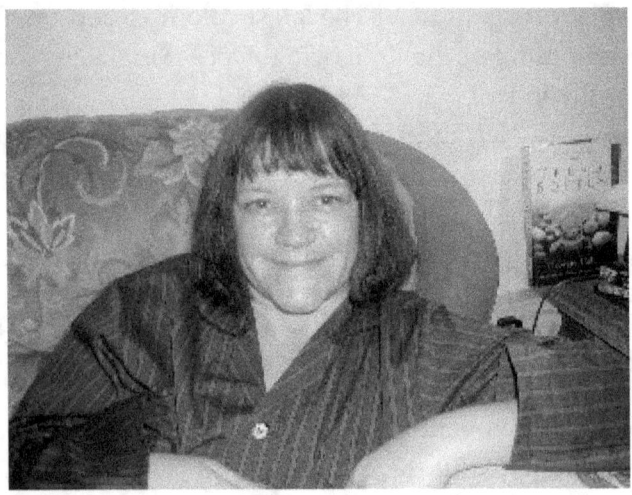

Lazing in my pj's with a shiny creamy face (am scared of wrinkles).

Monday 24th to Sunday 30th November 2003

Monday 24th November 2003

Weight 8 st 7 lbs (same)

Wonder what I will weigh today? Of course I am not getting anywhere with losing this 10 lbs I want to lose by Christmas (thereby taking me to under 8 st)...no, I am certainly not getting towards it. All in all it is because I am picking. I am eating fine in that I am mainly maintaining my weight, so should not complain, but I DO want to lose this last 10 lbs, it matters to me. And with only 5 or so weeks to Christmas at 2 lbs a week - constant - well, I had better make an effort, I know I can do it, I know I can....so as Steve (who works with Neil) once said "Just bloody get on with it then" Thanks StevieB!!!!!

Have taken to hiding the evidence (yep it has come to that again), you know, the WRAPPERS. Particularly the CHOCOLATE wrappers. Ho Hum.....I ran into the kitchen with said wrappers clutched in my hands (crunched up small in case I bumped into anyone (i.e. hubby or kids). Swiftly put them into bin and fled.

Cool work Cathy. Later that evening (last night) went to washing basket and what the.........there were the offending chocolate wrappers (how? how? When?).

Upon reflection the washing basket was right next to the bin (ok different colour but similar shape). The sad thing is...................I was not hiding the evidence from others , NO, why should my 2 kids bother and Neil would just say "Gimme some".........No ladies and gentleman, I was hiding those sneaky wrappers from myself and they bloody well came back to haunt me didn't they . A lesson to be learnt? Yes...move bin.

Still Monday (well...not quite true, it's 1.30 am Tuesday morning), yes I am still up. Went along to SW (of course) and am pleased to say I stayed the same weight, it even flickered briefly onto a lb loss. How many weeks to Christmas? So, an effort needs to be made. I would love a gorgeous red dress to wear this Christmas, oh and somewhere to wear it to! Please.

Tuesday 25th November 2003

2 small (emphasis on the small) apple and blackcurrant pies (i.e. Mr Kipling), a tin of low fat custard (emphasise the low fat) and a small (yes small, do remember I said small) piece of birthday cake. This is all the 'extras' I have eaten today, the unplanned extras. Mmmmm ok it is only Tuesday and the week is most definitely salvageable, so this is not my excuse to say "Oh bother...I've blown it so I might as well............" - no, I shall not do that. Tomorrow I shall, yes, eat better. Starting with brekky, yes a healthy weetabix n skim milk brekky, a salad and fruit for lunch and ermmmmmmmm can't decide about evening meal yet (too far away) and my exercise for tomorrow LINEDANCING.

I will not tear my hair out over what I have eaten, I will make the rest of the week a good week, this is what it is all about, doing your best and not giving up and moving on, I have eaten the stuff now and it's gone (ok most probably on my stomach or hips for the time being) but...but, never mind tomorrow is another day and there are 5 and a bit days till I get weighed again.

Thursday 27th November 2003

Is my dads birthday today, he is 60, we are off there after school today. I went Linedancing last night (have not been for a few weeks) and I thoroughly enjoyed it. Went to the Scouts Christmas Fair last night, had a mince pie and a coffee (yum) and won a teddy in the raffle. Actually I could choose a prize, on offer was chocolates and wine and a few other things. I thought about the wine of chocolates and decided to be saintly and got the cute teddybear. J was most cross with me for not getting the big box of chocolates. Afterwards I was cross with myself too!!!!

1st December to 8th December 2003

Monday 1st December 2003

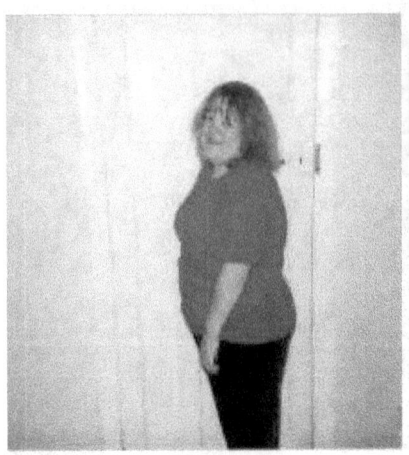 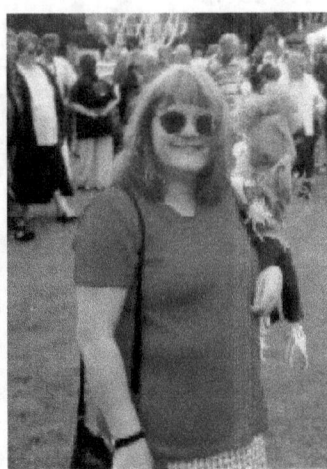

If I get whingey about my weight I must remember to look back at how I was before I lost the weight, it is easy to forget how much bigger I was. Nowadays when I feel fat I ought to look at these photos and when I am tempted to MEGA binge, I should also look at the photos........

> Weight today (here we go again)= 8 st 7 lbs
> (I stayed the same AGAIN)
> Lbs to lose (still) = 10+

Are we all getting in the Christmas mood? Already some of the houses round here are putting up their lights! I am going to a few Christmas type do's, namely

1. The SW one, which is being held at the hall we have the meetings in, each of us is taking in food (I will provide the cd player too.

2. The diabetic committee meal, which is being held at a hotel.

3. The college night out, we are all going to some pub/restaurant or other (Weatherspoons) and dunno after that, most will go onto a night club I expect (think I am too old!).

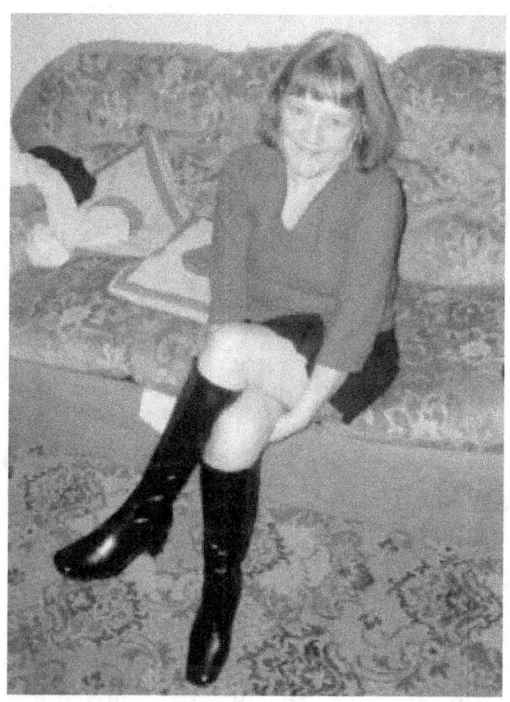

Wednesday 3rd December 2003

Oh I have really been eating too much and of the wrong things. I admit to having a WHOLE trifle the other night (I am sure it was meant for 4 people). I had several snickers bars this week....talk about binging. I have to stop.

Arghghghghhg where has the week gone?

Monday 8th December to Sunday 14th December 2003

Well, not long to go now for Christmas and already the parties have begun and I am certainly not going to make 7 st something for Christmas, but no matter. I am pleased with how I have managed to maintain my weight and hope I don't put too much on over the Christmas period!!

Note: Sunday 7th December

Arghghghghghgh I have been away on a diabetic weekend. How much have I eaten? TOO MUCH. And this is not to mention the alcohol!!!!! Set off Friday morning for Birmingham. Stopped on the way for pre-lunch (I was hungry) - got to the hotel 1.30pm booked in and realised evening meal was not till after 5.30 so we went to the pub next door for actual lunch. 7.30pm we finally got our meal (a 3 course Christmas dinner) but of course restaurants never give you too much do they!). Errrrrmmmmm lots of wine (got to get in the Christmas spirit). More wine. They did have a disco and I seem to remember dancing a lot, so got rid of a few calories there thankfully. BIG breakfast next morning - hey I was up at 6.00am bright and breezy - first person at breakfast! Started the course at 9 am, had lunch at 1pm and finished at 3.30 pm. Stopped for a meal on the way home. PHEW!!!!!!

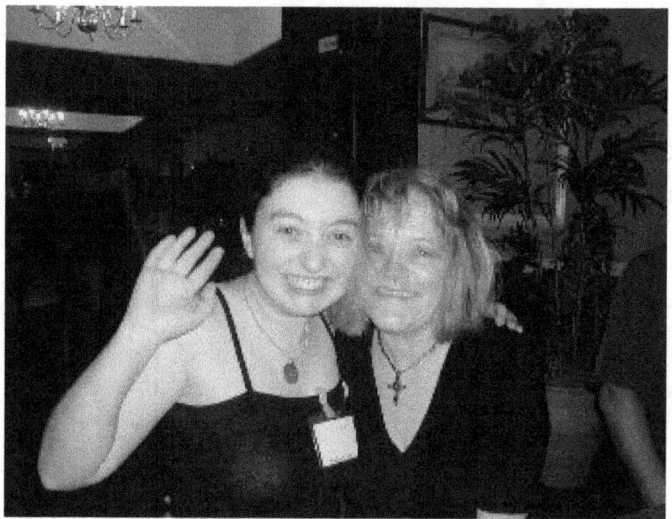

The weekend in B'ham, me and Cathy (yes same name) having been dancing those calories off! There was about 24 of us on the course.

Monday 8th December 2003

Now I have to face the music!! And if I have not gained any this week I shall 'eat my hat' because after all I have eaten and drunk, I should have gained at least 3 lbs, not that I want to of course.

Slimming World
Weight this week =8 st 7 lbs (119 lbs)
Weight last week was = 8 st 7 lbs
I lost/gained =NO, stayed the same
Lbs I still want to lose are = 10

I'll Eat My Hat if I had one! Can you believe that I stayed the same YET again? Yep I did. I even got on the scales a second time just to check, I was almost sorry I had not gained a pound, just a pound mind! Wouldn't want any more would I as I want to lose 10 more of them.

Thursday 11th December 2003

Bad habits, they are so easy to get back into aren't they!? I mean, take pastries for instance, the Cornish pasty type or mince pies or well anything with pastry......I could do without these, avoid them no problem. The thought of them never even entered my head. I could go into the bakers and huh phuh don't like them, don't need them can be so good not wanting them. Now along comes Christmas (arghghgh too many mince pies starting in late November) and a few dashes round the shops and OH what can I have for lunch? I know just one spicy beef pasty (or pastie however you spell it?). And now, well, I have had a few I can tell you, over the last few weeks.

But my body is strange and had allowed me to maintain my weight........another BUT and a big BUT, the weight has most definitely redistributed itself on my body and has chosen to settle on my stomach. My stomach is most definitely BIGGER. Not a good time of year to have a bigger (rounder) stomach.....all those clingy dresses.

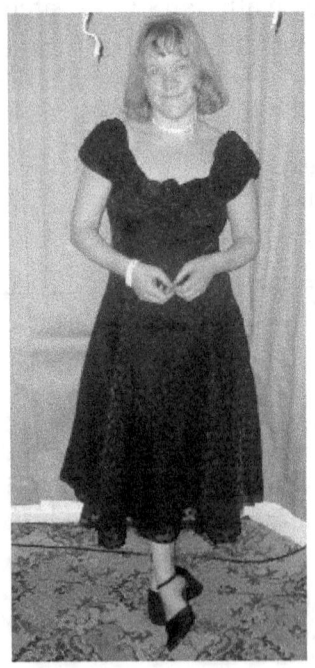

Here I am in the dress I am going to wear to my Linedancing party next week. We are having our usual class and all dressing up (party frocks) and taking food/alcohol along. I bought this 1950's dress from EBay and am going to wear this (but do my hair differently.)

Friday 12th December 2003

Did my text processing exam today (RSA 1), I did it or similar years ago but need to update. I think we all did well and hopefully we will all get distinctions. I am not aware of any MAJOR mistakes!

Sunday 14th December 2003

Had out DUK Xmas meal last night. It was nice. We had a 3 course meal and ok a fair bit of wine (not too much). I wore a strappy top and a long skirt but felt a bit self conscious about how I looked (in a fat mood). Today we (me and R) are off to my sisters for her little girls bday party.

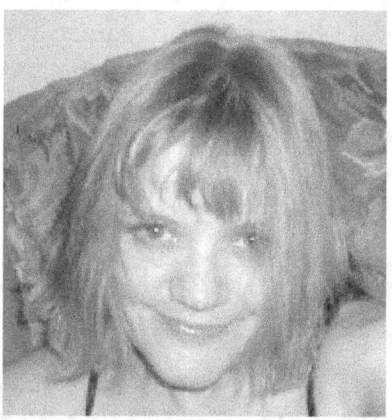

Trying to look ermmmmm sultry...no....sober? Yes! After the Xmas meal (back at home)

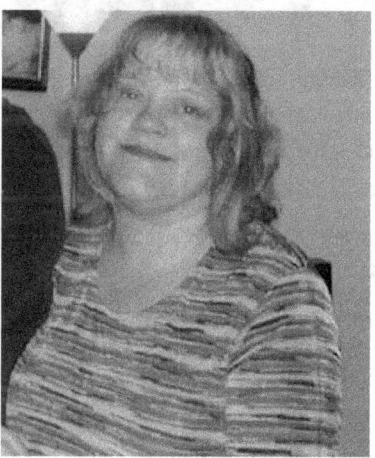

About 2 years ago holding my face up to disguise double chin!

Monday 15th December 2003

Monday 15th December 2003

Tonight is the Slimming World Christmas party, well, sort of a party. We are all taking food in and having some music. We have to get weighed first though! I shall have to wear light clothes! I have certainly gained weight this week, I can tell because things are tight on me that were loose.

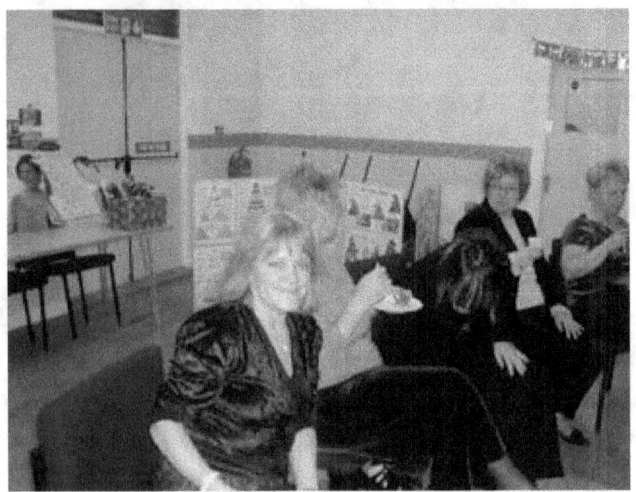

We had our SW party someone nicely or un-nicely made trifle and I just had to have 2 servings. And lots of other stuff - after all it was a Christmas party! Oh yes I certainly gained 2 lbs, was almost glad to really given all the stuff I have been eating and drinking lately.

Weight this week =8 st 9 lbs
Weight last week = 8 st 7 lbs
Gain= 2 lbs (yes my ermmm festive eating has caught up with me at last and there's still time to go before it is all over!!)

Thursday 18th December 2003

Went to my Line Dance class last night and we had our party. It was great fun, we played 'dance' games and of course did loads of dancing, had lots of party food (yum), most wore something glittery and I had my 50's dress on, ok I felt perhaps a little overdressed but nobody minded and that will be the only chance I get to wear the dress!!! It was a really nice night and I really enjoyed it.

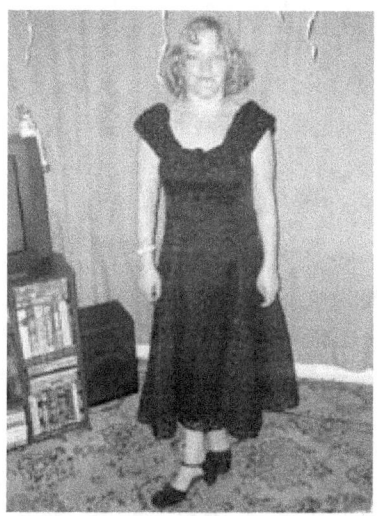

Ready for Line dance class party

I have my college get together (meal) on Saturday night (gosh all these do's - all this food! and ermmm alcohol!) Think I may gain a few lbs over Christmas. I had an exam yesterday (Word Processing level 1), will do level 2's in all exams after Christmas. Am feeling a little lumpy around my middle (all these mince pies) and have taken to hiding my middle again (with cushions etc when I sit down). I know I have gained TOO much when I hold it in and it doesn't hold in!!!!

Maybe I ought to wait till after Christmas to get serious about dieting again? Yes???????

Monday 22nd December to Sunday 28th December 2003

Merry Christmas Everyone

Mmmmm not a good time to be dieting eh! I am doing Christmas dinner at my mother-in-law's, I am doing all the cooking.

> Weight = don't know
> Weight last week = 8 st 9 lbs
> Lbs still to lose = about 10 or 12

Didn't get weighed this week but know I have gained weight cos stomach is so much flabbier.

Monday 22nd December 2003

Yes I am getting weighed tonight, just a weigh-in, no meeting. I was 8 st 9 lbs last week and only have 1 lb to spare, just one pound that I can gain then I will be OVER my target weight ARGHHHHHHHH. I was hoping to be under 8 st 5 lbs for Christmas so I COULD safely put some on...............but it was not to be. I am HOPING to stay the same tonight (fingers crossed)

Am not sure if I am going to get weighed tonight as Neil and I are going shopping when he gets home from work. I will try to get weighed even if I pop in very quickly. I am sure I am over my target now though. Had a good night at the college do, WAY too much wine (enough said!).

Well I didn't go and get weighed, I went shopping instead and did loads of walking (feet are killing me now). Had to eat so went to McDonalds (unfortunately) and had a chicken burger thing and fries.

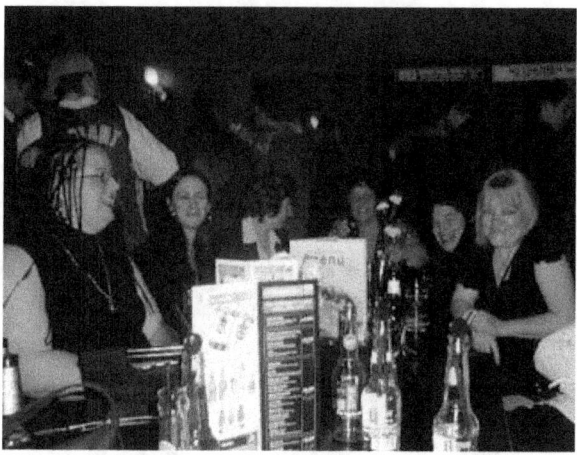

At my college Christmas party

Tuesday 23rd December 2003

Want to be lazy today but I still have about 8 presents to get. I bought the turkey yesterday and have a few other little bits and pieces to get.

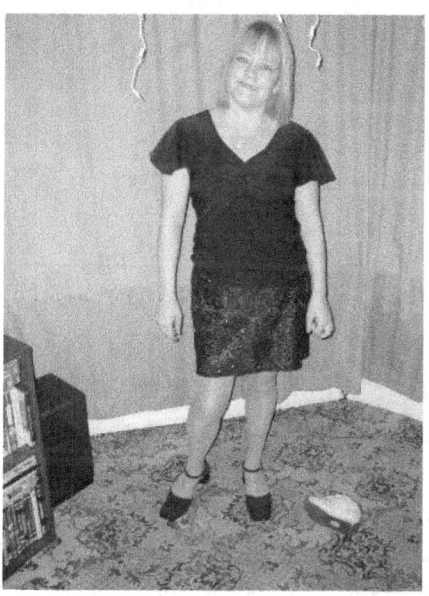

This was taken just before I went out on my college Christmas 'do' on the 20th December

Am starting to feel very flabby and fat round my tummy area so I will HAVE to get back on the diet plan after Christmas.

In February I go to work in a local newspaper for 7 weeks (part of my college course). I am really looking forward to doing this (if a bit nervous). It is my local paper called The Wirral Globe (you can see the online version of it). Everyone on my course has to do a placement, you had to choose and contact your own (where you would like to do your work experience).

My sister Cheryl is in hospital, her baby is due about 14th Jan and she has high bp so they have taken her in...this is her first baby.

Wednesday 24th December 2003
CHRISTMAS EVE

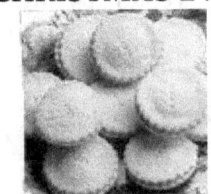

MMmmm mince pies

You just have to eat don't you? I mean, mince pies, cream, sweets and all that. Not that I have had a lot of course?!

My sister had her baby last night weighing 4 lbs 6 ounces....tiny. We are now trying to get the kids to go to bed.....no such luck so far (ok is only 5 pm but...) hehe no actually it's 8 pm.

25th December 2003
Christmas Day

Ohhhhh I have eaten too much!! Here I am at my mother-in-laws. I had gone to church in the morning in a nice skirt but put on loose jeans for Xmas dinner (just as well!).....here I am trying to hold stomach in!

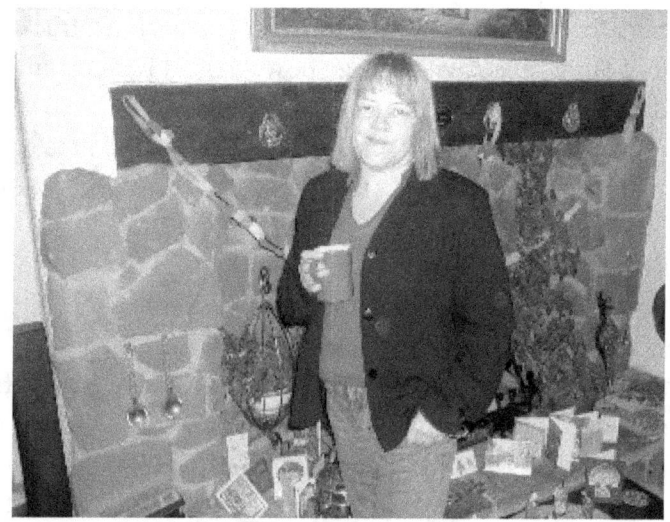

I think I may have gained about 8 lbs

26th December 2003 Friday BOXING DAY

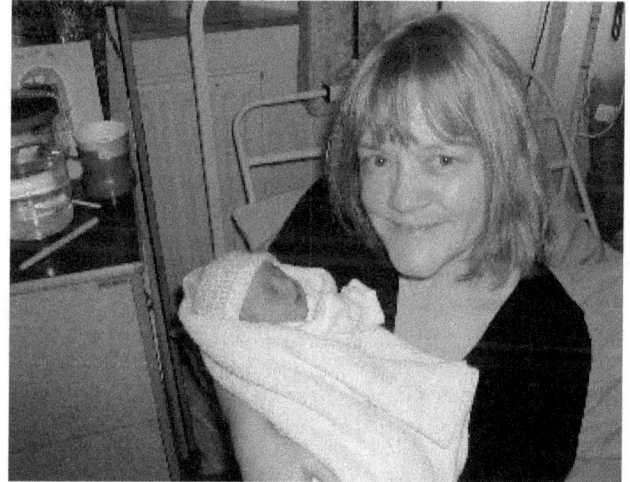

We went to see my sisters new baby (they have not decided on a name for her yet). She is sooooo tiny and beautiful.

Saturday 27th December 2003

Am feeling so disgusted with my stomach really I am. It feels bloated and BIGGER. I am going to face the music on Monday and go and get weighed. Part of me feels like giving it a miss for one more week (so I can get back on track first) but no, I am going to go and see how MUCH I have gained on Monday. It is just a weigh-in, no meeting.

I have got the ski-walker out in the bedroom...it is up and ready for me to get using. After all I paid £80+ for it and have hardly used it....so, I think it is about time I used it, say every day for ermmmm s short time!!!!!

Good thing is we are out of sweets and chocolate. We never really do anything special for New Year (not my favourite holiday of the year).....though I do have a bottle of wine for Neil and I to have a drink New Years Eve (we shall aim to watch a good film or something). It is going to be difficult to get back into proper eating and not snacking and picking (i.e. eating sweets!).

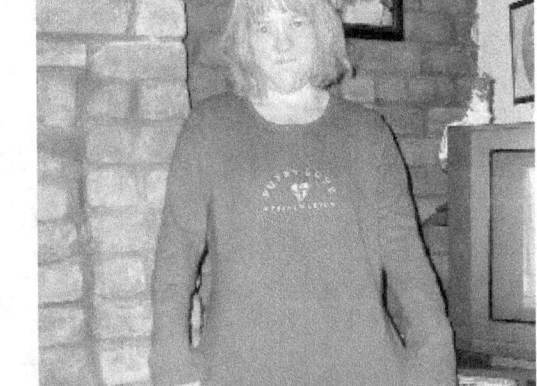

In my pyjamas feeling FAT. Ok, I do not look so fat but my flab is hidden by the baggy pj's really it is. If I were to be wearing something slinky and clingy I would look awful.

Sunday 28th December 2003

I think I will try and stick to the diet today. We do not have anything planned for the day. I believe the shops are open again (the supermarkets) and we may go and stock up on some healthier foods. I actually did 20 minutes on my Railwalker last night....am not aching yet!

My clothes are getting tight!

Monday 28th December to Sunday 3rd January 2004

Monday 29th December 2003

I face the scales TODAY!

Nearly time to go and get weighed. I have truly made an effort today and stuck to the eating plan.....thought I had better make a start. I guess (predict) that I have gained 6 lbs (taking me to ermmmm about 9 st 1 lbs)?????? If I am very lucky it will only be about 3 lbs gain......I HOPE.

WEIGH-IN

Weight this week = 8 st 11 lbs (123 lbs)

Gain of = 2 lbs

Lbs I want to lose = Altogether 13 lbs

I am pleased to say I only gained 2 lbs. I have a new book from Slimming World, this will motivate me to get back on track. I also bought the latest Slimming World magazine and am going to sit down and read this later with a cup of tea.

Tuesday 30th December 2003

I am feeling very determined. I actually stuck to the plan all day yesterday - all day. Though I was very hungry in the evening so we ate omelettes (these are free on the plan).....yes we were eating omelettes about 11pm last night. It's funny how when you decided to get SERIOUS you get hungrier.

Neil has also started the 'diet' and is following the Slimming World Plan. I think it is important we have all the 'free' foods in so that when he gets hungry he can eat these. He managed to get through yesterday (just about)! I had to throw out some cheddar biscuits he was tempted by (after having eaten almost the whole lot the day before.

Arhghghghg scary photo. Me on the mini trampoline that Neil got me for Christmas (it arrived today). I shall be bouncing up and down for a few weeks!! Mmmm how long will the novelty last I wonder?? Actually it seems like a good buy, I like it (so far after a few bounces and jogs) and the kids like it. It is easy to store away and pretty sturdy. Unfortunately Neil has to lose about 25 kgs before he can use it, but I cannot see him happily jumping up and down on it anyway!

Hopefully all of this will help me lose the last of my weight. I am back to my Line Dancing class on Wednesday evening (next week/next year!).

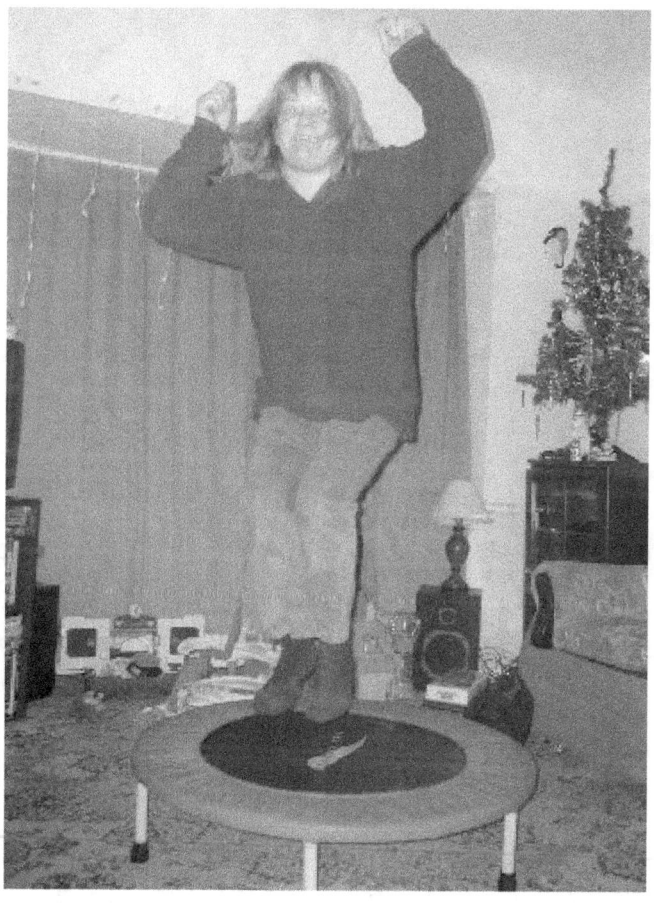

End Of Volume One

Appendix

1. Cathy's Cartoons

I have drawn these cartoons using Photoshop. I am not the world's best artist!!! Please feel free to copy any of these if you wish (a link saying where you got them would be nice). Also if you like them, let me know, also if you think they are rubbish let me know (but be nice/kind!) Thanks..............

When I am asleep it is easier to diet!!!!!!!!!!!!!!!!   **I hide my tummy with cushions, bags and kids.**

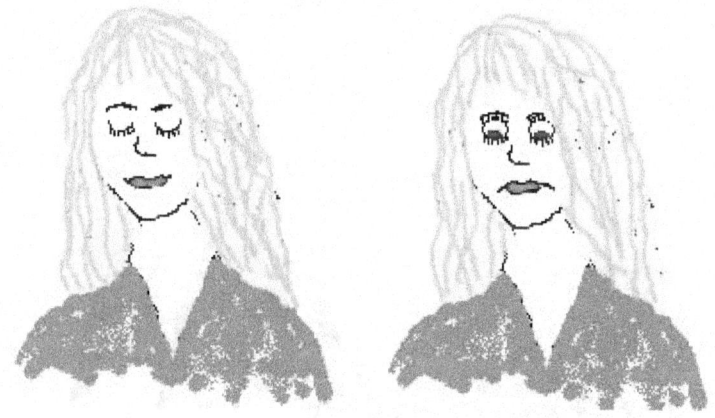

Mmm..I should not be eating this!!!   **Weigh-in tonight, before I eat of course!**

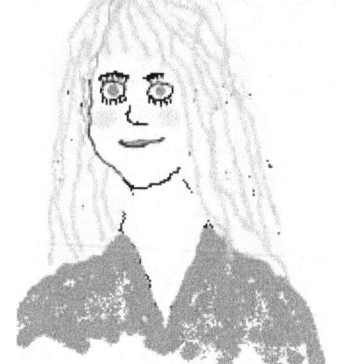 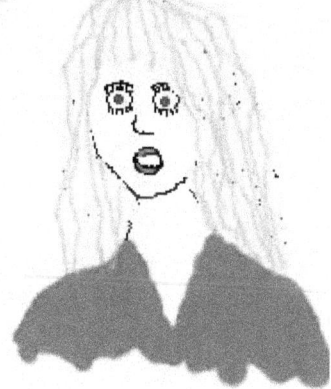

The Coffee Diet

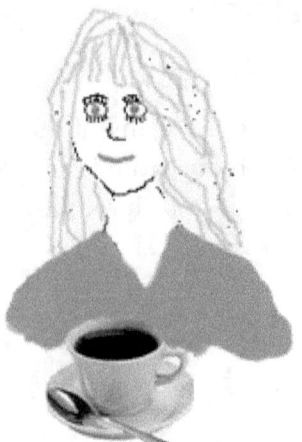

I may have lost
my weight but
I still have bad
hair days !!!!!!!!!!

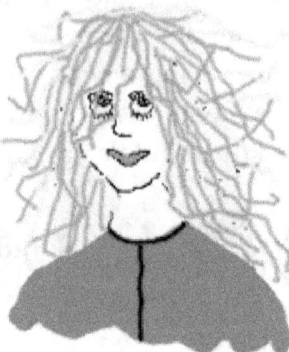

I am sure high-neck
sweaters make me look
like I have a double
chin.

It's Halloween!
I get to wear black,
which is so slimming.

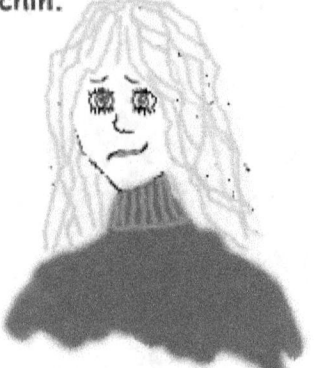

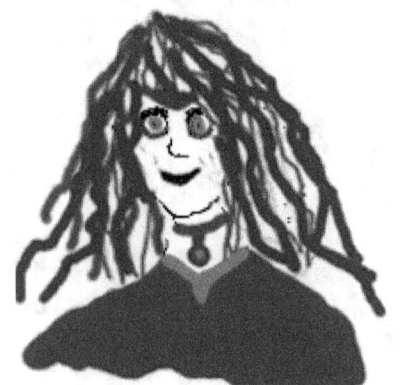

A fringe can hide many things: Spots, frown lines, tired eyes etc. It can look sexy when used correctly!

Sometimes my stomach is a bit too demanding. It asks for seconds and even thirds!

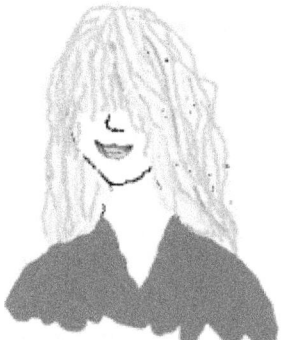
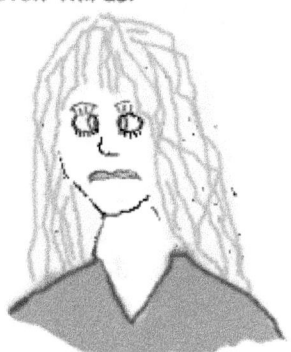

2. Holiday Photos

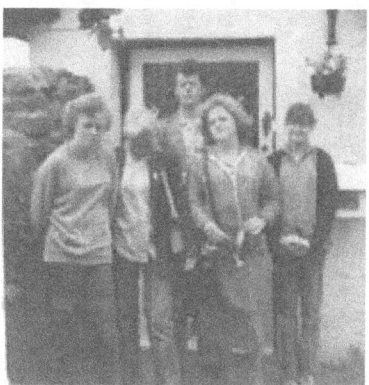

Summer 1980 (me in the orange skirt) Weighed about 7 st 10 lbs (108 lbs)

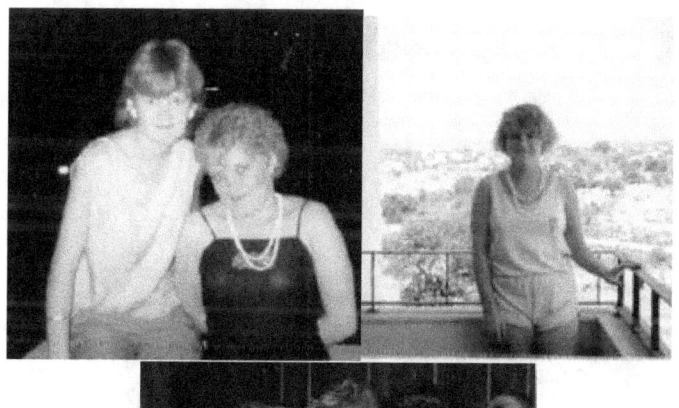

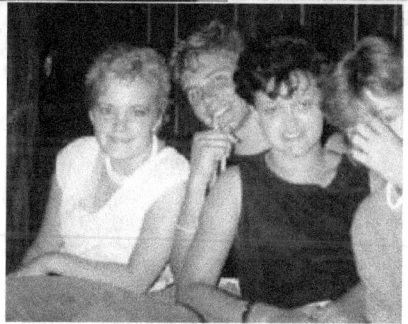

(Above)Summer 1983/84/85. Weighing about 8 st (112 lbs)

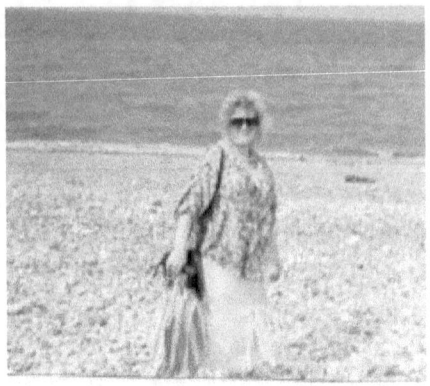

Summer 1990 weighing about 9 st (124-6 lbs)

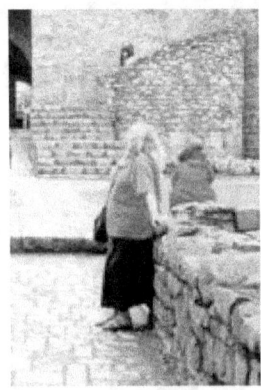

Summer hols 1999, I weighed about 11 st 12 lbs (166 lbs)

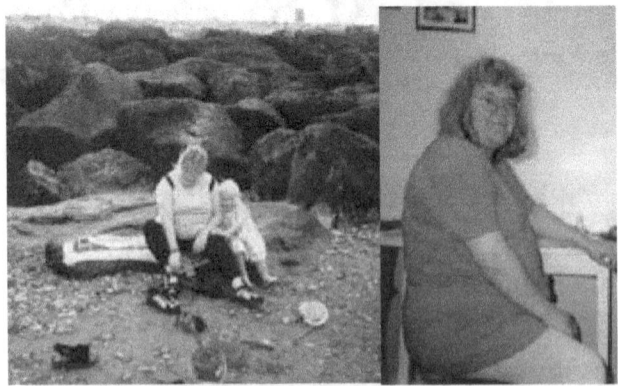

Summer 2000 weighing about 12 st (170 lbs)

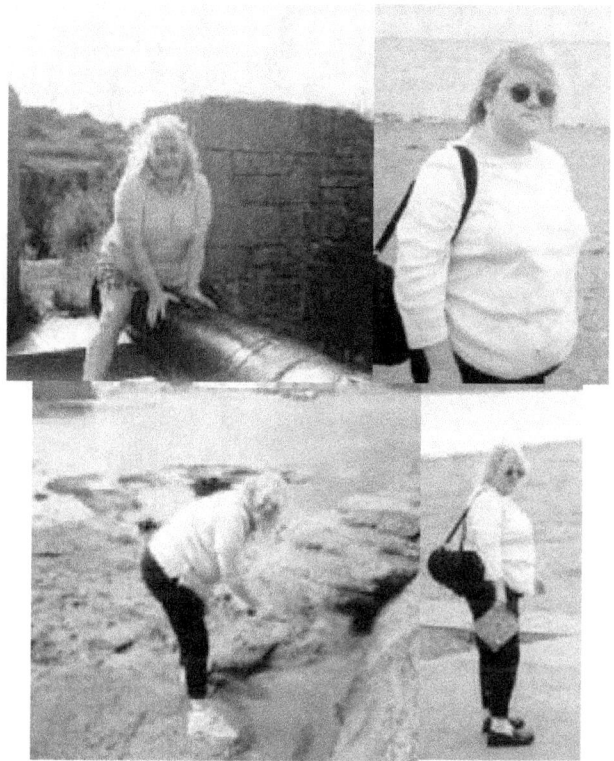

(Above)Summer 2001 weighing 11 st 7 (161 lbs)

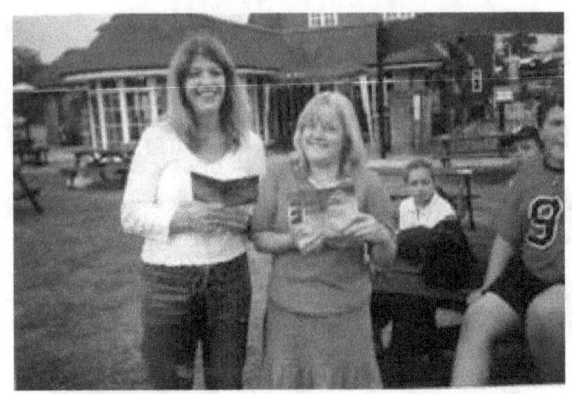

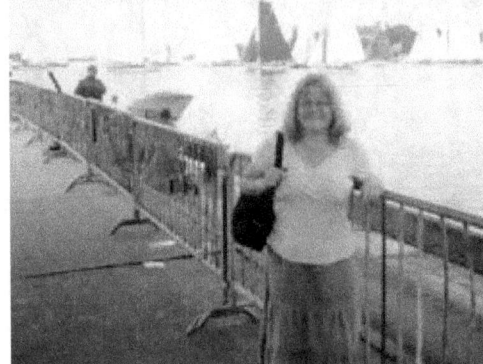

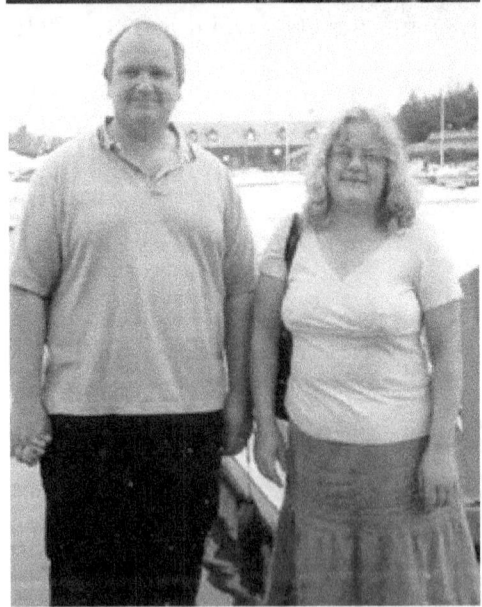

(Above)Summer 2002 weighing 10 st (140 lbs)

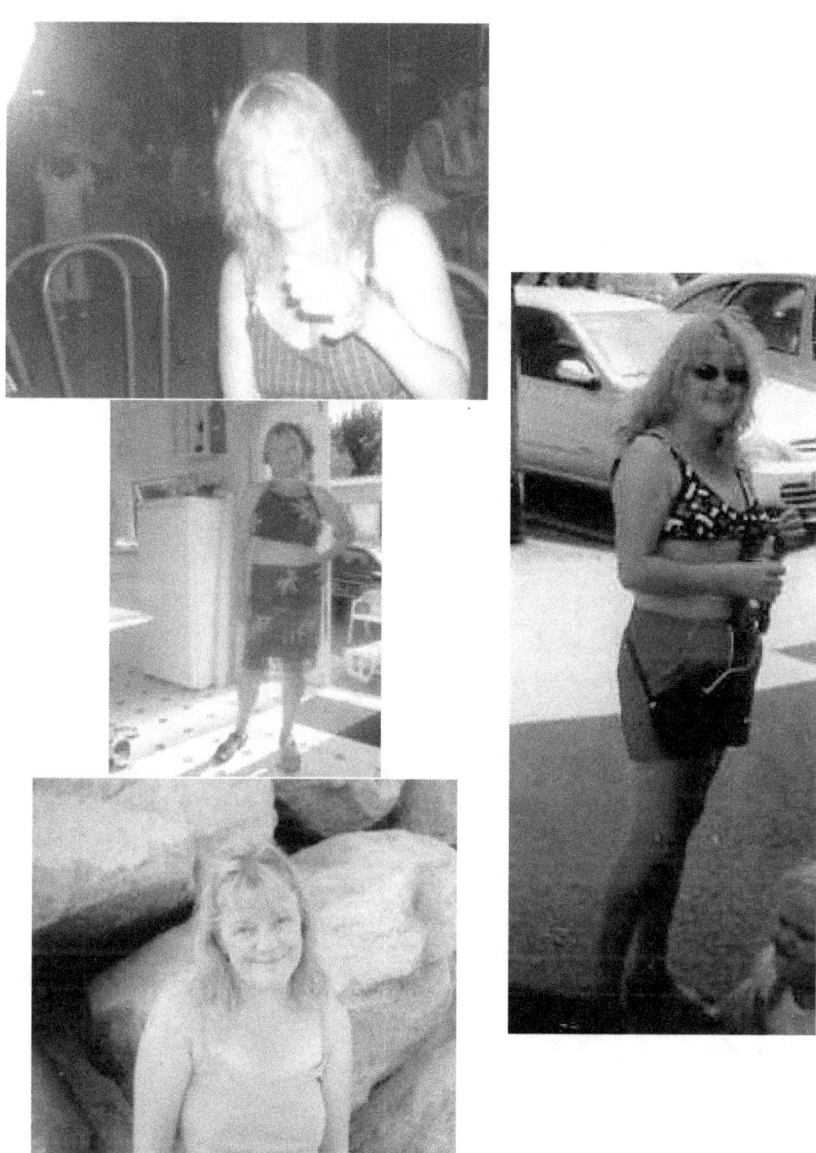

(Above)Summer 2003 weighing 8 st 5 lbs (117 lbs)

3. Wouldn't It Be Loverly Diet Song

Words By Cathy Davies/Music by Frederick Loewe

All I want is a chocolate bar
Oh so sweet but it won't go far
Lick hands, yum yum, nice taste
Oh wouldn't it be loverly

All I want is a chocolate cake
Mmm to eat and so nice to bake
Warm hands, full tum, nice taste
Oh wouldn't it be loverly

I know that if give in
that I will get so fat
I know that I have to so resist this loverly stuff

All I want is a nice dessert
Surely one, well it wouldn't hurt?
Fold hands, big tum, no waist
it wouldn't be so loverly
Loverly

All I want is a nice flat tum
Shapely legs and a curvy bum
Slim arms, trim thighs, oh please
Oh wouldn't it be loverly

All I want is a gorgeous dress
To look slim and not a mess
I know I can do this
Oh it can be so loverly

I know that if want to be like this

I have to try
Now I know that I can be so very very good

All I want is to now succeed
I will do it now you will see
So slim so trim that's me
Oh it will be so loverly
Loverly
Loverly
Loverly
Loverly

NB: Hubby is SO fed up with this tune cos I have been playing it 100's of times so I could make up the words to it!

www.ingramcontent.com/pod-product-compliance
Lightning Source LLC
Chambersburg PA
CBHW070846290526
45795CB00001B/4